Living with Brain Injury

A Guide for Families

The Second Edition

Richard Senelick, MD, &
Karla Dougherty

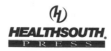

HEALTHSOUTH.
PRESS

This book is not intended to replace personal medical care and/or professional supervision; there is no substitute for the experience and information that your doctor or health professional can provide. Rather, it is our hope that this book will provide additional information to help people understand the nature of head injury and its effects on its victims and their families.

Proper treatment should always be tailored to the individual. If you read something in this book that seems to conflict with any of your doctors' or health professionals' instructions, contact them. There may be sound reasons for recommending treatment that may differ from the information presented in this book.

If you have any questions about any treatment in this book, please consult your doctor or healthcare professional.

Also, the names and cases used in this book do not represent actual people, but are composite cases drawn from several sources.

© 2001 by HealthSouth Press
One HealthSouth Parkway, Birmingham, Alabama 35243

Published by HealthSouth Press

Library of Congress Catalog Card Number: 2001132779
ISBN-13: 978-1-8915-2509-4
ISBN-10: 1-8915-2509-3
First HealthSouth Printing
10 9 8 7 6 5 4 3
HealthSouth Press and colophon are registered trademarks of HealthSouth Printed in Canada

THE FACTS ABOUT HEALTHSOUTH

HealthSouth Corporation is the nation's largest physical rehabilitation healthcare provider with over 100,000 patients being treated in its facilities every day.

The HealthSouth network includes rehabilitation hospitals and acute-care medical centers, as well as outpatient rehabilitation, ambulatory surgery, and diagnostic imaging centers. Some of its diverse services include the treatment of brain injury, sports injuries, spinal cord injury, stroke, pain management, and such diagnostic services as mammography, magnetic resonance imaging (MRI), nuclear medicine, and ultrasound.

HealthSouth Press has been created to help patients and their families understand the ramifications of their injury or illness. All of its books are created to help families learn how to cope with life's unexpected changes. And, above all, each book is designed to show, in compassionate and intelligent terms, that you, the reader, are not alone.

ACKNOWLEDGMENTS

We would like to thank Tony Tanner, the former Executive Vice President of HealthSouth, for his support and leadership in the creation of the HealthSouth Press. Thanks, too, to Brad Hale, Gerald Nix and Gray Richardson of HealthSouth for their help in seeing this manuscript through to fruition, as well as the entire production and art staff of HealthSouth Press.

We would also like to thank Hal Hoine, Ph.D., and Elizabeth Bilderback, M.S., from the HealthSouth Rehabilitation Institute of San Antonio Department of Rehabilitation Psychology for their help in educating patients, families, and ourselves about the effects of brain injury. Without them we cannot imagine how we would be able to care for the patients and their families.

DEDICATION

This book is dedicated to the patients and families who have had to endure the tragedy of brain injury. It is through them that we have learned so much, both intellectually and emotionally. They endure on a minute-to-minute and hour-to-hour basis those things that we all hope we will never have to face. We have never walked in their shoes nor had to sit in their chairs, but we hope that our collective experience in dealing with brain injury rehabilitation will help families adjust to a new way of life — as well as deal with the difficult issues and challenges that arise on a daily basis, We are constantly amazed at the strength and adaptability of the human spirit and the day-to-day strength that is shown to us by the families of our brain-injured survivors.

CONTENTS

THE IMPACT OF THE BRAIN IN TODAY'S WORLD

• *Jimmy calls himself the "walking wounded." He works as a messenger delivering packages and letters to offices and apartments throughout downtown Orlando. He likes to wear a tie, even when the weather is hot and humid. He looks perfectly presentable; people who pass occasionally smile hello. But if, say, a woman stopped and asked him for directions, Jimmy would first look at her blankly, then, he'd start to stammer. He might even get angry and spew out a string of obscenities. What this woman and others didn't realize, at first, is that he had a severe brain injury years ago. Jimmy's scars are invisible.*

• *Arlene was riding her brand new bicycle down the hill near her house. She'd walked, run, ridden, and sledded down that hill so many times in her young life that she could close her eyes and instinctively know she had reached the bottom. That's exactly what she did this spring day. Unfortunately, she couldn't see the broken tree limb sitting in the middle of the road. She hit it at full speed, flew over the handle bars, and hit her head. She is still in a rehabilitation hospital, recovering from her brain injury.*

• *Sam loved his new position. As vice president in charge of sales for a major corporation, his responsibilities were enormous. But, then again, Sam always did have a great deal of energy. He always had time to listen to his subordinates' complaints and suggestions. He met his deadlines and was always one step ahead of the competition. In short, Sam was a one-man dynamo of executive capability, and it was no secret that he was being groomed for the corporation's top spot. But all this was before his accident. A two-car collision on the interstate left Sam befuddled, confused, and angry. Although he suffered only a mild head injury, the damage was enough to sabotage his managerial talents. He could no longer lead — a fate Sam refused to acknowledge. By not accepting this, Sam became an unhappy, bitter alcoholic.*

These are only three short stories, three vignettes of people whose lives have been irrevocably changed because of a brain injury. Unfortunately, they are not alone. Nor are their accidents isolated ironies of life. A staggering 2 million people suffer from mild to moderate brain damage every year, with 17% suffering from serious brain trauma that results in neurological deficits and loss of consciousness. But there's more: Only 5% of them get the help they need.

ONE LIFE TO LIVE

As late as the 1970s, 90% of all brain-injured patients died. Today, thanks to an abundance of medical advances, higher-quality technology, and improved emergency care, more and more people are surviving — not only military vets who sustained brain injuries in battle, but ordinary people with ordinary lives. Add the fact that contemporary Americans take more risks — from bungee diving to mountain climbing, from driving cars at breakneck speeds to pursuing the brass ring at any cost — and the evidence is undeniably clear that brain injury has indeed become a "Silent Epidemic."

CAUSE AND EFFECT

It's a fact: A brain injury can occur to anyone at any time. But there are some specific arenas that put people more at risk:

• *The young between the ages of 15 and 24 always take more 'daredevil' chances* — with motorcycle, bicycle, and car crashes causing more brain injuries than any other mode...

• *But the figures climb back up again after the age of 70,* with most brain injuries the result of falls.

• *Bicycle accidents are becoming one of the major causes of head injury* — with over 1,300 deaths each year. But wearing a helmet can drastically cut down on the risk.

• *The causes of brain injury vary according to geography.* In our car-oriented San Antonio, Texas, location, motor vehicles are the number-one culprit. In some cases, firearms and assaults account for most of the brain injuries. In cities where there's a great deal of construction and development, industrial accidents cause the most damage.

MIND OVER MATTER

In many ways, the brain is our most vulnerable organ. An injury to the head doesn't heal the same way the heart, or the liver, or a broken leg does. It isn't a matter of "staying off your feet for a few weeks" or "getting plenty of rest" or "taking two aspirin and calling the doctor in the morning." Brain injury affects who we are; the way we think, act, and feel. It can change everything about ourselves in a matter of seconds. And it can create havoc in the people we love, our family and friends, who are suddenly faced with a disabled stranger with:

• *Cognitive dysfunction...* including memory loss, perception and comprehension difficulties, and deficits in attention, organization, problem solving skills, and reasoning.

• *Physical impairments...* including partial paralysis, spasticity, lack of coordination and balance, and swallowing difficulties.

• *Behavioral problems...* including over-aggressiveness, depression and mood swings, violence, and lack of impulse control.

But all is not bleak. The medical and technological advances that have kept brain-injured patients alive have also developed better and more successful treatments.

THE "RE" FACTOR

Brain recovery often means extensive rehabilitation — retraining and relearning that requires time, consistency expertise, and a structured, secure environment. In fact, without rehabilitation, the patient may stop far short of his potential. Here's proof: In a study of severely brain-injured young adults with serious cognitive and emotional disturbances, 50% of those who received rehabilitation were found to be productive three-quarters of the time, as opposed to only 36% of those who did not receive treatment. Ultimately they were not only less emotionally disturbed than those head-injured young adults who did not go through rehabilitation, but they also did better on memory and learning tests. Other studies of severely brain-injured patients who had received rehabilitation found that many of them were able to become useful members of society, if they had support.

These results are not surprising. It is only in a rehabilitation setting that a patient will have the most advanced equipment and most comprehensive care. And it is only in this setting that a family can get the education they desperately need to cope with the day-to-day problems that crop up in brain injury — and to truly help their hurt loved ones.

But perhaps the most compelling reason for rehabilitation is its goal: independence. With successful treatment, a brain-injured patient may regain at least some of his ability to:

1. Live, work, and enjoy life in our society.
2. Redevelop social and family relationships on a more equal basis.
3. Participate within the community.

However, proper rehabilitation doesn't come cheap. A person with a moderate brain injury can conceivably spend more than $100,000 in treatment. The figure can zoom literally into the millions for severely brain-injured survivors who need long-term care.

Fortunately help is at hand. The United States government has recognized that brain injury is indeed a serious problem nationwide. Congress had declared the entire '90s "The Decade of the Brain," appropriating $15 million to the dual fields of brain injury rehabilitation and brain injury prevention. As we head into the first decades of the 21st century, brain injury research continues to be at the forefront of scientific and medical funds allocation; brain injury and brain safety continue to make the news in all media throughout the world.

The insurance industry, too, has discovered the benefits of rehabilitation in the bottom line: Every dollar used for brain injury rehabilitation saves up to $35 in future medical costs.

Yet, despite this important financial and public recognition, there is no denying the pain of the individual family, the individual victim — and the high cost of brain injury in both emotional and practical terms. There is, after all, no price tag on loss, no "discounts" on the turnabout of fate. But there is hope.

And that's where this book comes in.

BRAIN INJURY: A GUIDE FOR FAMILIES

We have been involved in the field of head injury rehabilitation for many years. In our work at HealthSouth RIOSA, we have seen countless incapacitated brain-injured patients become functioning members of society. Together, we long felt the need for a clear and helpful guide for families who are thrust into the world of brain injury — a book that would not only contain all necessary information, but offer reassurance as well. Thus *Living with Brain Injury: A Guide for Families* was born, a book that not only addresses you, the family members, but medical professionals who are just now embarking on a career in head injury rehabilitation. Now the demand for this book in the United States and around the globe has created the need for a second edition — one that includes more up-to-date information and one that addresses the concerns of families in the new millennium.

Within these updated pages, we will take you on a journey through the brain. You will discover how the brain works, and why. We will explore the many varied and complex symptoms that come into play when the brain is injured. Step by step, we will show you the rehabilitation process, including the new theories of neural plasticity and constraint therapy, as well as offer sound advice on choosing the best rehabilitation hospital for your loved one. And, most important, we will pinpoint how you can help a brain-injured survivor in the best and least stressful ways — for both of you.

We know there is life after brain injury. After reading this book, it is our hope that you, too, will believe this to be true.

AN ANATOMY LESSON

"What a piece of work is a man!"
William Shakespeare, Hamlet, Act II, Scene 2

Picture this scenario: It is a bright summer day, a perfect Sunday in which you have nothing better to do than sleep, or think, or spend time with someone you love. As you prepare a picnic, you tuck in amid the sandwiches and fruit that new book you've been dying to read. You and the one you love drive out to the country to an empty meadow. You lay out your blanket and eat your food and talk of romance. Settling down, you lean back against the cool trunk of a spreading apple tree. You close your eyes; you feel the cool breeze on your flushed face. You sleep... and wake up with a start and an exclamation of pain. "Ow!" you say, rubbing your forehead. You look down by your leg and see the culprit: an overripe apple,

If your name was Newton, this situation might lead you to the discovery of gravity. But if you are a mere mortal like the rest of us, you have just learned from an experience.

You have used your brain.

We are not often aware of our brain, of its unflinching attention throughout every second of our days — and nights. But think of it: In the above scenario, you anticipated a pleasant day. You organized and planned your picnic. You discussed love and life and felt the joy of real contentment. You ate your food; you swallowed your cider; you fell asleep. And, when your nap was interrupted, you perceived and understood how the apple fell from the tree.

You learned not to go to sleep under any more apple trees. You stored this information and made it a part of your memory... Yes, all these examples of how your brain was involved, intertwined, and incorporated in your day!

The fact is, in many ways, the brain is a marvel. Although it weighs less than three pounds, it controls, initiates, stores, and comprehends every facet of our lives — from enabling us to automatically perform the proper steps for brushing our teeth to giving us the capability to feel the beauty and pathos of a concert symphony.

Under normal conditions, we don't give our brains another thought. We simply live our lives — until tragedy strikes. Then a brain injury occurs, and the functions of the brain we take for granted can run amok. Depending on the location and severity of the injury, we feel its effects cognitively, behaviorally, physically or, more typically, as a combination of all three.

But unless you understand how a normal brain functions — how its different areas communicate with each other and with other parts of your body — you won't understand what happens when it is injured. Before you can discover what's wrong, you have to know what's right in...

THE ANATOMY OF THE BRAIN

Although it might look like a damp, frequently used sponge, don't let appearances fool you. The brain consists of a complex network of billions of nerve cells called neurons. It has very specific locales, with each one responsible for a particular function. It can store tremendous amounts of information and, when it is working properly, there is nothing in our manmade world that can compare to it, not even the most sophisticated computer.

The scarecrow in *The Wizard of Oz* bemoaned, "If I only had a brain." Well, if he did (and, as we all know, he only *thought* he didn't), it would be set up something like this:

1. The Peripheral Nervous System

Remember those Visible Man and Visible Woman dolls, the clear plastic ones with the veins and arteries all on display, or the visible humans you can download on the Internet? Well, in the same way veins and arteries are intricately spread throughout the body, so are peripheral nerves. From the nerve endings at your fingertips to the nerves in your muscles, from the nerves entwined in your organs to the nerves attached to your spinal cord, all are in play, all carry messages to the brain. The hot stove you touch, the ice-cold drink you taste, the tack under your bare foot — all these sensations, or stimuli, travel toward the brain to elicit a response. Then the brain sends a message back, and you quickly withdraw the sore foot. Without the brain's interpretation, the pain or the thirst-quenching feeling would be meaningless; you wouldn't feel or think anything of these sensations at all. Think of the peripheral nervous system as a messenger service, traveling throughout the "city" of the body to pick up and deliver a specific action, thought, or sensation.

2. The CNS

No, it isn't a discount chain for men's fashion. CNS stands for the Central Nervous System or, to be more exact, the spinal cord and the brain. The CNS is the master control, the chief of all the nerves. The spinal cord is the first stop; it is a go-between, a relay station that connects the peripheral nervous system with the brain. Messages go up and down your spine, so to speak, delivering stimuli to the brain that must be interpreted, and then the brain's reply travels down to the rest of the body — responses to speak, move, listen, gesture, show emotions, or any combination of these.

3. The Brainstem

Traveling up the spinal cord, we find the next stop on the "upper management floor": the brainstem. It consists of three areas, the:

Medulla, which is as basic as you can get. Here are the life-sustaining controls for blood pressure, heart rate, and breathing in and out.

Pons, which is a bridge linking the medulla to the higher, more evolved areas of the brain. Here, too, is the reticular formation. It is a conglomeration of nerve fibers, helping to control muscle tone, reflexes, wakefulness, and mechanisms to keep you alert and ready to react to change.

Midbrain, which gives you, and lower animals, eye muscle control and more "reticular formation" action — from staying more alert to keeping your reflexes honed. It is also a bridge between the brainstem and the cerebellum (coming up next).

The entire brainstem is attached to the spinal cord by thick nerve fibers.

4. The Cerebellum

Travel behind the brainstem and you'll find the cerebellum, the area of the brain that regulates all your movements, balancing and adjusting every step and every stance. Its also a wonderful "traffic manager," smoothing and coordinating your movement and your speech muscles. *Basal ganglia,* located higher in the cerebrum (see page 13), are its sidekicks, helping the cerebellum to modulate and modify all of your movements.

5. The Diencephalon

You'll find this area right above the brainstem and right below the majestic, higher-functioning cerebrum. It's the true gateway to higher thought and emotional depth — and not just because of its location. Why? Because it's home to the *hypothalamus* and the *thalamus* — two key players in the brain game. All sensory information, from the ridiculous to the sublime, must first pass through the thalamus, which works like a switching station in a railroad yard. Here, your mother's meat loaf recipe will be delegated to your memory storage tank in the temporal lobe. At the same time, the brainstem starts you salivating in anticipation of dinner. A Walt Whitman poem might find a place in your memory right next to the meat loaf, but its words also travel to the limbic system (coming up next), which controls your emotions. It might make you soar. Or as the poem ricochets back and forth from the emotional limbic system to the more intellectual areas of the brain, you could find yourself contemplating the ironies of life.

In short, the thalamus is a beehive of activity, sorting out messages and deciding which areas of the brain get what.

As you might have guessed from its spelling, the hypothalamus is its cousin. No bigger than a pea, it rests right below the thalamus. But don't let its small size mislead you. The hypothalamus' influence is vast. From appetite control to sexual arousal, from thirst to sleep, from balancing body temperature to keeping hormonal secretion intact, the hypothalamus does all of these and more. And, because of its close proximity to the emotional limbic system and the intellectual cerebrum, it also plays a role in regulating your emotions, motivations, and moods.

6. The Limbic System

Anxiety. Joy Anger. Elation. None of these emotions works in a vacuum. Thanks to the limbic system, the interlocking structures of nerve cells that run between the diencephalon and the intellectual cerebrum, you can literally feel and express your emotions. Because the limbic system lies so closely to the cerebrum, your feelings are very much tied to your thoughts, perceptions, and attitudes. Without the limbic system, you might cry or laugh, but it would signify nothing. With an intact limbic system, you can have real emotion, filled with color and depth. You can feel the glory of that summer day in the apple orchard. You can feel embarrassed when the apple falls on your head. And because of the link between the limbic system and the intellectual cerebrum, you can remember this day not just as a series of events but as a look at the past.

7. The Cerebrum

This is the area of higher-functioning thought, memory, and perception. As you might expect, this is the largest part of the brain, and it is home for several interrelated areas.

The hippocampus and the amygdala are responsible for emotion, memory, and thought. The hippocampus sits directly in the temporal lobe of the brain; it is connected to all your senses — and to the limbic system. Its sister, the amygdala, is nestled within the limbic system itself. Together, they can trigger a rush of emotions and coinciding thoughts. Let's go back to the apple orchard for an explanation:

It's now the cold of winter. You are hungry, but your refrigerator is bare except for some slowly rotting apples. You look at them; you smell their pungency. Thanks to the hippocampus, these senses connect you back to that summer day in the orchard, a memory that has been sitting in storage. These vivid memories now flooding the hippocampus trigger the limbic system into action. The system's amygdala comes to attention, rushing the flood of memory through the limbic network, flashing its own emotional images of that summer picnic into the nostalgic brew.

You remember. Your thoughts return to that day, and you can feel the emotion of the day.

MORE TO "C" IN THE CEREBRUM

The *cortex* is the gray lining that covers and clings to the cerebrum. Think of it as a stretchy, wrinkled blanket made of billions and billions of nerve cells that covers... the *cerebrum* itself, the chunky gray and white matter of the brain. Between the two lie all your thoughts, movements, and stored memories, all that you learn, understand, and communicate. Here is where you are most human — and most vulnerable when it comes to head injury.

The *corpus callosum* is similar, in many respects, to an interstate highway. Rich in nerve cells and fibers, it connects...

... the *right* and *left* hemispheres of the brain, Think of a line going down the middle of your brain, dividing it into two perfect mirror images, a right and a left side. Although pop psychologists have turned "right-brain" creative thought and "left-brain" logic into a magic formula to "find" the real you, in reality, both hemispheres work together, communicating via the corpus callosum. Here's an example of the right and left-brain hemispheres in action:

You see somebody you'd like to know better. You approach the person and start up a conversation. That's your left brain in action. Perhaps you slowly drawl out your "hi." Perhaps you look right into the other person's eyes for dramatic effect, or perhaps you make a joke such

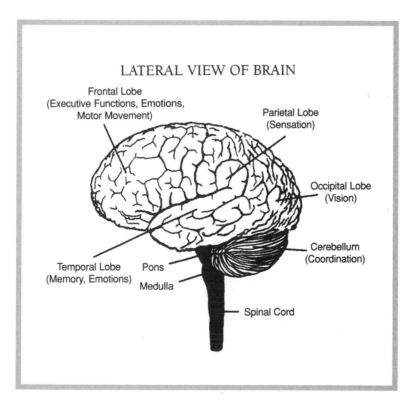

LATERAL VIEW OF BRAIN

Frontal Lobe
(Executive Functions, Emotions, Motor Movement)

Parietal Lobe
(Sensation)

Occipital Lobe
(Vision)

Cerebellum
(Coordination)

Temporal Lobe
(Memory, Emotions)

Pons

Medulla

Spinal Cord

> ## HEADLINERS
>
> *A study printed in the* New England Journal of Medicine *proved, beyond a doubt, that bicycle helmets save lives. For one full year, Dr. Robert S. Thompson and his colleagues studied bicyclists who had sustained head injuries while bicycling. Their results? Ninety-nine cyclists had severe head injuries — only 4% had been wearing helmets. Those who wore helmets reduced their risk of head injury by a full 85%! Since most bicyclists are children, helmets can be considered a wise investment in everyone's future.*
>
> *How to get your children to wear helmets? An evaluation of a community-wide helmet campaign in Seattle found that helmet wearing increased 14%. But in Portland, where no such program existed, helmet use only increased from 1 % to 3.6%. Get your schools, your communities, and your local government to act. Public campaigns work!*

as, "We have to stop meeting like this." Whatever "line" you choose, it's your left brain that gives you the ability to speak and use language, but your right brain gives what you say its dash of color.

Your left hemisphere is also more responsible for all your other language abilities — from reading to calculating and writing.

Your right side controls your visual memories, your ability to draw or copy, play music, or dance. It's also the right side that allows you to see the bigger picture, the consequences of your life further down the road.

When brain injury occurs in only one hemisphere of the brain, the result is seen in the opposite side of the body. A damaged left brain could result in paralysis on the right side of the body, and vice versa. Emotional differences will also be noticed: Injury to the left hemisphere can commonly cause depression. But the same injury in the right hemisphere could actually make a person unaware of his deficits.

MOTHER LOBE

Not only is your brain divided in half, but each half has four lobes, each with a different function:

The _frontal lobes_ are, of course, in front. They are, in many ways, the commanding officer of the brain. Here you will find controls for impulse, motivation, social abilities, expressive language, and voluntary movement; you'll also find the ability to retrieve memory from storage. These lobes also control your "executive functions" which include the abilities to plan and organize, to stay focused, to make decisions, and set goals.

Unfortunately, the frontal lobes are very vulnerable to brain injury. The traumatic results? You might not be able to say what you mean. You might not be able to generate any new ideas. Your attention might be scattered. You might lose control over your impulses and become aggressive, abusive, and coarse.

The _temporal lobes_ are just behind and below the frontal lobes; they are nestled above our ears. They are as vulnerable to brain injury as the frontal lobes. They hold the bulk of your memories, both recent and from the distant past. Here, too, is the home of the hippocampus and its bounty of emotional thoughts. The temporal lobes also control your ability to understand language and appreciate music. The temporal lobes are the processing house for your perceptions; they put "law and order" into incoming information, sequencing it, and making sense out of what you hear.

Damage to the temporal lobes can mean that you will have trouble remembering things you'd done just an hour ago. You might not be able to perceive what someone means. The Mozart you hear might sound like cacophony.

The _parietal lobes_ sit above the ears, near the back of the brain. You might call these the "sensitive" lobes because they control your sense of touch, and they play a major role in your academic abilities, including reading comprehension and deciphering spatial relationships.

Damage here can hurt your ability to physically feel and recognize an object. You might find yourself unable to read even simple sentences. You might find yourself unable to distinguish an apple from an orange; to you, both appear equally strange.

The _occipital lobes_ are literally "the eyes in the back of your head." They are responsible, purely and simply, for sight. If you injure your occipital lobes, you can become blind.

These, then, are the parts of the brain itself. But no man is an island, and no brain stands alone. In fact, it floats like Jell-O® in what we call... cerebrospinal fluid. This is a clear liquid that surrounds the brain, nourishes it, and protects it much as an airbag might protect a passenger in a car. This fluid also fills the open spaces or ventricles of the brain. Six times a day, new fluid replaces the old.

The _cranium_ is the skull that completely contains and protects the brain. But there's more to this floating, encased "cocoon" — and its lining of membranes — that, in his book, *Clinical Neuroanatomy Made Ridiculously Simple*, neurologist Dr. Stephen Goldberg calls "P.A.D." for short. In actuality, these membranes, or meninges, are:

1 The *pia*, a thin lining that literally hugs the brain.
2. The *arachnoid*, a spider weblike lining that is sandwiched between the pia and...
3. The *dura*, which rests right up against the bone of the cranium. It is strong and durable.

The P.A.D., which surrounds the entire central nervous system, provides further protection for the brain. But when head injury occurs, the P.A.D., too, can be damaged, with blood hemorrhaging and collecting beneath or between the linings, severely complicating the initial injury.

Knowing the different areas of the brain and how they function is one thing, but understanding how they communicate with each other and with the rest of your body is another. Let's take a look at the message-relay system.

LINES OF COMMUNICATION

Remember your summer day in the orchard? The cool breeze, the delicious picnic, the pain when the apple fell on your head — all these facts had to be sent to your brain for decoding, deciphering, storing, and responding. Messages had to go back and forth throughout your brain, from your limbic system to your frontal lobe, from your right hemisphere to your left, not to mention the ongoing, continuous messages for breathing in and out coming from your brainstem.

Scientists now know that these messages are conducted

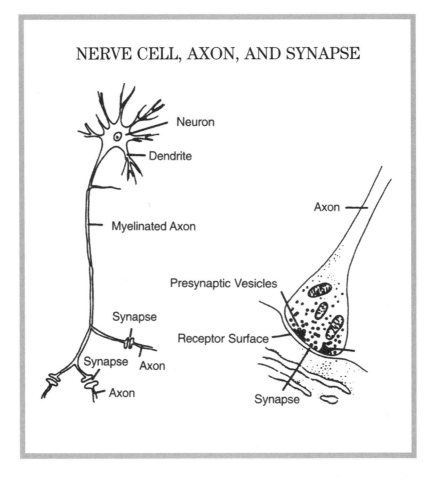

NERVE CELL, AXON, AND SYNAPSE

Neuron

Dendrite

Myelinated Axon

Axon

Presynaptic Vesicles

Synapse

Receptor Surface

Synapse Axon

Axon

Synapse

from nerve cell (neuron) to nerve cell via both electrical and chemical conductors. Fortunately, it's not as complicated as it sounds. Listen:

An electrical impulse carrying, say the "ouch!" of pain from the falling apple, travels through a *neuron*, from its outlying *dendrite* tentacles to its central *cell body* and out again along a thin passageway called an axon. But as

---

HEADLINERS

Axons are covered with an insulation called myelin, which serves almost the same purpose as insulation on your electrical cords at home. This insulation protects the axons and also helps conduct electricity at a much faster rate, sending electrical messages at a fast clip. But when the axons are stretched, electricity cannot be conducted as quickly or efficiently. This may result in many of the physical, cognitive, and behavioral problems encountered in brain injury. If the axon heals, all may eventually be well. But if the axon is severed or torn, it may not be able to repair itself, and the symptoms may be permanently disabling.

"ouch!" gets to the end of the *axon*, there's a space called a *synapse*. The next neuron lies in wait, but the electrical charge can't cross the synapse. "Ouch!" would become history at this point, except that the electrical impulse then triggers the release of a chemical, a *neurotransmitter*, which crosses the synapse to a receptor on the next cell. This starts the electrical conduction down the new axon. "Ouch!" continues on its way until it reaches a new synapse, where the electrochemical process once again takes place. (See illustration on page 20.) In fact, countless chemical neurotransmitters lie like silent wallflowers at the synapse, waiting for that one "Mr. or Ms. Right" to supply them with an electrical spark. In other words, only one specific electrical impulse will activate a specific neurotransmitter that will jump across the synapse and activate the electricity waiting in the new cell.

Now picture this activity occurring all over your brain at a fast and furious pace, relaying message after message to its different areas, deciphering, storing, and shouting commands all at the same time. Excuse the pun, but it boggles the mind how accurate, how attuned, and how precise the human brain remains, day after day!

From the need to yawn after your picnic lunch to the desire to sigh as the warm breeze hits your face, from the "ouch!" of the fallen apple to the "ah" of a kiss, the messages transported through your brain are as varied and unique as you are. But there is one basic theme to almost every chemical message that crosses over a synapse, as crucial a rule to remember as one plus one equals two:

NEUROTRANSMITTERS CAN EITHER INHIBIT OR EXCITE ACTION, BUT MOST OF THEM INHIBIT

Yes, it's true. Most neurotransmitters soothe the savage beast. Left to your own devices, you might respond to "ouch!" with a grand slam throw of the apple in the vicinity of a nearby window — or your unlucky partner. You might further be inspired to add a few choice curses, followed by a temper tantrum in which you trampled the apple into mush.

Instead, the message you receive from your brain is, "Calm down," "stay cool," or even, "forget the apple. Go home, think about your day, and discover gravity."

Unfortunately, most of these inhibitory messages originate in the frontal lobes, which, as we have already mentioned, are especially prone to injury.

This is almost the end of the anatomy lesson. But there

is one more rule to remember about the brain: The whole is indeed much greater than its parts. Each of the various components, from the lobes to the hemispheres, from the neurotransmitters to the cerebrospinal fluid, work together to create you — your unique personality, your unique attitudes, intelligence, and emotions. This "uniqueness" makes brain injury all the more devastating when it occurs. By understanding how the normal brain functions, you will not only understand what happens when things go wrong, but you will be able to grasp how varied and individual the resulting symptoms can be.

Yet as singular as each case ultimately is, brain injury happens in only a few basic ways. In fact, that's the subject of the very next chapter. Read on...

CHAPTER TWO

WHEN BRAIN INJURY OCCURS

"I used to think this kind of thing only happened
on TV or in the newspaper — not to people I know
and love. And especially not to me..."

A brain-injured patient at HealthSouth RIOSA

Michael had always wanted to be an attorney. And at 35, his dream had come true. He was a prominent attorney for a topnotch Louisiana law firm. Michael worked hard — too hard, if you asked his wife. When his old college buddy told him about a great deal on a one-week fishing excursion in Canada, even his wife urged him to go. He agreed. It was time for a little R & R.

Unfortunately, it was rainy and windy their first two days in the wilderness. The third day proved the same. Impatient and suffering from cabin fever, Michael and his buddy decided to go out on the lake anyway. But the weather only got worse. Halfway across the water, the boat began to pitch and roll. Michael fell and struck his head on the side of the boat.

His friend managed to get him back to the cabin. Michael had been unconscious for only 10 seconds, but he remained dazed for five minutes more. He then complained that he had a splitting headache; he felt dizzy and nauseous. But his symptoms didn't seem that bad, and he didn't want to spoil the trip, especially when the next day proved to be sunny and warm.

Yet when he returned to the law firm, Michael still felt dizzy and nauseous, and had an almost continuous headache. To add to his problems, he also found it difficult to concentrate on his work. He couldn't look at a single file for more than 5 or 10 minutes; the words would start to blur together.

Michael decided his problems were caused by his eyes. He just needed new glasses, he thought. He went to his optometrist, who could find nothing wrong.

Michael's wife was getting upset. For the past few weeks, he had been acting peculiar. Formerly calm, caring, and stable, he had suddenly become a stranger. He was apathetic. He ignored the kids, and he had absolutely no interest in sex. He was easily frustrated and irritated. When the optometrist failed to find a problem, Michael's wife insisted he see their internist.

The internist referred Michael to a neurologist, who took a series of diagnostic X-ray tests that all proved negative. Later, however, Michael underwent neuropsychological testing that revealed that he had suffered a mild head injury, caused by his boating accident.

A rehabilitation program concentrating on his attention and memory deficits and his emotional responses helped Michael in only a few short months. Within three months, in fact, he was back on the job, a successful attorney who still worked too hard, but who made time for family vacations... on land.

It was several weeks before Michael's brain injury was recognized for what it was — a situation that's more common than you might think. Brain injury can be difficult to diagnose for several reasons:

• Its symptoms are easily labeled as something else — migraine headaches, overwhelming stress, or, in Michael's case, the wrong eyeglass prescription.

• The resulting injury includes symptoms that may be as individual as the victim himself.

• Not everyone who has an accident suffers from brain injury. Another fisherman might have hit his head and suffered nothing more than a minor bump that went away within a day.

• Brain injuries are sometimes so microscopic that, as with Michael, they are difficult to detect, even with the most

---

HEADLINERS

Myth: If you've injured your head, doctors will identify it immediately.

Wrong. Head injuries can be "invisible." The amount of damage can't always be seen, even with a CT scan or a more advanced brain scanner called MRI (Magnetic Resonance Imaging). Why?

• There are so many nerve fibers in the brain — billions and billions, actually — that it's difficult to pinpoint which are damaged and which are not.

• The damage, as in diffuse axonal injury, can be widespread, affecting many different areas of the brain.

• Microscopic damage can't always be picked up, even by the most advanced diagnostic tools. Yet microscopic damage can pack a wallop. It can cause problems such as depression and confusion, which are made worse when its victims are told "it's all in your head."

advanced diagnostic tools. Yet small does not necessarily mean minor. Even the most microscopic brain injury may cause problems.

Despite the masks that can conceal brain injury from both patient and physician, certain universal characteristics act as clues.

HEADS UP

From strokes and tumors to Parkinson's Disease, your brain can be injured internally, without any outside intervention. But a discussion of these diseases belongs in a different book. The brain injuries we're addressing here are the ones that are traumatic — that is, caused by a fall, or a car accident, or a bullet, or even a boat on a stormy lake.

These injuries occur suddenly and without warning, interrupting what until then had been a normal development.

A simple truth:

The brain governs and regulates everything that makes a person human from the way he thinks to the way he acts, from the way he walks to the way he feels. Thus damage to the brain may leave him significantly changed.

Like Michael, a calm person might suddenly become irritable at the slightest provocation. He might become self-destructive, reaching for drugs or alcohol to ease the pain. He might cry at the slightest provocation.

When you consider that damage may be contained in one specific area, creating very specific symptoms, or it may be widespread throughout the brain, creating many unpredictable symptoms, you get an idea of how complex a brain injury can be.

SKULL DUGGERY

There's nothing like an imposing skull to send goose-bumps down a horror fan's arms, but there's more to its shape than just the scare factor. Look again. It's completely smooth. But if you were to run your hands along its interior, you would notice "innards" that are rough, bony, and ridgy, especially the area near your forehead and ears where your frontal and temporal lobes reside. Under normal conditions, your brain is happily bobbing in its sea of cerebrospinal fluid. But if your head hit the steering wheel, if you fell off your motorcycle head-first without a helmet, if you slipped on a staircase and tumbled down 12 steps, your brain — along with the rest of your body — would get shook up. It would bounce and jiggle within its skull home, hitting and rehitting those bony ridges around your forehead. And which areas of the brain would most likely hit and rehit this ridgy skull zone? None other than the higher-functioning frontal and temporal lobes, which hold those thoughts, actions, and motivations that make you human and unique.

PUSH AND PULL

This starting-stopping movement of our brain when it is injured has a name. It's called an *acceleration-deceleration* injury.

Let's say you are driving along in your car (acceleration) until it crashes into a tree and comes to a sudden stop (deceleration). This abrupt acceleration-deceleration movement causes the brain to strike the bony ridges of the skull, resulting in bruising, hemorrhaging, and even stretching or tearing of the axons in the brain. The brain

---

HEADLINERS

"I evaluate myself in relationship to the way I was prior to the accident and in comparison to other victims. The characteristics of brain injury vary from individual to individual, and the length of time since the injury is also a major factor. About three years ago, I did something very funny which was an example of the type of poor judgment encountered by head injury victims. I called the police to report a lost cereal bowl!

"Head trauma isn't like mumps or measles, which go away after you get them — it's with you for life. You just compensate for it. It's a long, rocky road. My lifetime goals are to excel as a father, a son, and as husband. My accident didn't change these — it put an emphasis on them... "

— James Blakely,
a brain-injured person
from Tucson, Arizona

(Reprinted from "First Person Accounts" from the Brain Injury Association, Inc.)

---

can also be bruised by a direct hit on the skull. Sometimes the impact causes the brain to move in the opposite direction, such that a blow to the front of the head causes a bruise in the back of the brain. This "backhand" phenomenon is called a *coup-contrecoup* injury.

A COMMON FRONT

Most traumatic brain injuries result from acceleration-deceleration action, and many of these head injuries result in frontal and temporal lobe bruising, which we call *frontotemporal contusions.*

These bruises can create short- or long-term memory loss, as well as language deficiencies in either comprehension or production. Damage to these lobes can also affect motor skills and coordination, visual perception, attention, behavior and more — all symptoms that we discuss in depth later in this book.

Adding insult to injury, there's more to brain damage than frontotemporal contusion. In addition to the bouncing ball of the brain hitting the "concrete" wall of the skull, stretching and tearing can occur — with serious repercussions.

DIFFUSING THE ISSUE

The brain does not stand alone. As we mentioned in Chapter One, its stem is attached to the spinal cord by a cluster of thick nerve fibers. When the head is struck and the brain twists and stretches within the skull, these nerve fibers are pushed and pulled in all directions. In fact, when the head is hit with any sort of force and the brain is violently shaken, the nerve fibers (axons) within the brain can be stretched. A fall; a car crash that thrusts a victim through a shattered front window; a vicious fight — all these can cause widespread damage throughout the brain. Called *diffuse axonal injury*, this condition may result in a coma that can last anywhere from a few days to a few months or years, especially when the brainstem nerve fibers are sheared. Because this area of the brain affects our very survival — from breathing to staying awake — damage here can be long-lasting and devastating.

A SWELLED HEAD

Unfortunately, brain injury is a painful example of the whole that's greater than its parts. It's more than sheared nerve fibers and an acceleration-deceleration injury. A bruised brain can become swollen — the worse the damage, the more it may swell. Although that might not sound so serious in light of everything else we've discussed, *swelling can be one of the major reasons for brain damage.*

Think of it. When you bang your foot, say, against the coffee table, it will swell. Similarly your brain will swell when hit. But there is a crucial difference: When your foot swells, it's easy enough to go without shoes for a few days. But your brain is encased in a finite amount of space. When the brain swells, it has no room to expand within the confines of its rigid skull. Instead, *intracranial pressure* builds and builds, damaging even more nerves and causing even more pain.

It is crucial that the swelling be treated quickly. Unless medication and proper treatment to reduce the swelling are given in the acute-care hospital, the pressure will continue to build, damaging more and more nerves. *(We'll discuss brain swelling and other secondary physical symptoms of head injury in more detail in Chapter Six.)*

But wait. There's still more. Brain injury is not only categorized as a possible frontotemporal contusion, a diffuse axonal injury, or a swelling. It's also diagnosed according to whether the injury is open or closed...

AN OPEN BOOK

A bullet wound... a shard of glass... a forceful blow with a heavy instrument... any of these can penetrate the brain, damaging both it and its surrounding skull, causing both a skull fracture and brain injury. Any accident involving an outside force that penetrates the head is called an *open head injury*, which has its own problems, because:

- Pieces of skull, skin, hair, and debris are literally pushed into the brain, creating bruising, bleeding, and swelling. Add a skull fracture, and there is even more pressure on an already weakened brain.
- The foreign matter that has entered the brain makes infection a great risk.

CLOSED QUARTERS

Damage from a *closed head injury* is seemingly invisible. Because the skull is not penetrated, everything appears intact. But inside, the damage begins as the brain pounds against the bony ridges of the skull. Like Michael, who hit his head against the boat, some people with closed head injuries don't receive a proper diagnosis for several weeks or even months.

The majority of head injuries are closed. And a closed head injury is vulnerable to diffuse axonal injury and swelling. From memory loss to dizziness, there may be some sort of neurological impairment — sometimes temporary, but other times a permanent fact of life.

You now know how the brain gets damaged. But that's still not enough. For physicians to diagnose the extent of a brain injury, they must determine the degree of injury that has taken place. For them to create a helpful, constructive rehabilitation program, they must go beyond the diagnostic categories of open or closed, diffuse axonal injury, or frontotemporal contusions. That's exactly what we'll discuss next.

CHAPTER THREE

DEGREES OF INJURY

*"Life is what happens while you
are making other plans."*
John Lennon (1940-1980)

***MYTH: Someone with a mild head injury will
always come out of it fine.***

FACT: Not necessarily. In about 15% of people, the effects
of mild injury may linger, which can affect a person's thinking process, motor control, and mood.

***MYTH: Someone who has had a severe brain injury
will always be a "vegetable" — and would
be better off dead.***

FACT: Not so. Every day science offers new research
and technology to help people live longer and better. We have seen some survivors of severe brain
injury progress from a deep, long-lasting coma to
an ability to recognize loved ones, laugh, join a
conversation — and contribute to society

MYTH: No one ever gets better without rehabilitation.

FACT: Not always. Many people actually do have some
spontaneous recovery which occurs without rehabilitation care. However, rehabilitation can prevent
medical complications and provide social, physical,
cognitive, and vocational skill training, all of which
can help recovery flourish and reach higher levels.

HEADLINERS

C IS FOR CONCUSSION

The word concussion is more complicated than you might think. On one hand, a concussion is defined as a temporary loss of neurologic function. But on the other hand, there doesn't have to be a loss of consciousness at all.

Further, one brain injury predisposes a person to the cumulative effects of subsequent brain injuries. A concussion might be the "ding" a third baseman hears for 5 to 10 minutes after he's been hit by the ball, or the fumbling of a football quarterback who gets progressively worse after every tackle. The effects are cumulative — as with the "punch-drunk" fighter who can no longer hit a moving target or even see it. Brief episodes of memory loss may add up to periods of amnesia or permanent memory impairment. (See the next chapter on mild head injury.)

Perhaps it's because brain injury involves the brain and the vast mysteries of the mind. Perhaps it's because the psyche is involved — the undefinable characteristics that make a person not only human, but unique. Perhaps it's because the injury occurs so swiftly, so traumatically — and can change life so irrevocably. Perhaps it's because so many areas of a person's being are affected — from the way he thinks — to the way he walks across a room, from the way he conducts himself in public to the way he reads and writes. Whatever the reasons, traumatic brain injury is clouded with half-truths, myths, and erroneous beliefs.

This makes sense — brain injury is difficult to accept and to understand. It can be extremely complicated, involving so many diagnoses, so many treatments, so many symptoms But there's room for optimism.

CLASSIFIED INFORMATION

Despite the confusion, medical professionals and scientists have helped separate the wheat from the chaff. Categorizing the different ways that the brain can become injured helps doctors determine the severity of a head injury and predict what the outcome will be. Mild head injury, the most common, will be discussed in the next chapter, but it's important to be familiar with the other degrees of injury

Classification #1: Moderate Brain Injury

This is more than a minor, slight bump in the head. It means the person has been unconscious from 15 minutes to 24 hours. It also means that he may be hospitalized for several weeks. Once the crisis has passed, he will probably be transferred to a rehabilitation hospital. The amount of time he will spend there will depend on the extent of his disabilities and on his progress, but it's likely he'll call the rehab hospital "home" for an extended period of time.

Symptoms vary from individual to individual, but moderate head-injured survivors may suffer from:

- Tremors or balance problems
- Paralysis
- Seizures
- Memory deficits
- Poor judgment and problem-solving
- Weakness
- Lack of coordination
- Language problems
- Perceptual difficulties
- Behavioral problems

Some sobering news: A study by Drs. D.W Corthell and M. Tooman discovered that as many as two-thirds of survivors with a moderate head injury are unable to go back to work one year after the injury.

Classification #2: Severe Brain Injury

In severe head injury, brain damage will be deep and diffuse, and the victim will be poorly responsive for at least one day. He will have physical deficits; he probably will have muscle coordination problems, and he may be paralyzed or spastic. Rehabilitation is always required.

Severe head-injured survivors may go back to work after intensive vocational training, but usually in a reduced capacity. Many such victims must remain in the care of their family or a supported living environment.

Classification #3: Catastrophic Brain Injury

When physicians cite a "persistent vegetative state," they are usually referring to the consequence of catastrophic injuries. Here, victims will be in a deep coma for months, years, perhaps forever. They might have sleep and wake cycles, but this is not true awareness. They must be fed; they cannot speak; they probably do not understand anything that is said to them. Unfortunately, even at the top rehabilitation hospitals these patients may demonstrate only modest improvement. However, an adequate trial of rehabilitation is in order to get the person properly seated, splinted, and positioned before deciding on long-term placement.

These are the three types of brain injury, but the most common type of brain injury needs a chapter all its own. Read on...

HEADLINERS

Sarah Brady had to have been incredibly angry when her husband, James Brady, was shot during an assassination attempt on then-President Reagan's life. But both she and her husband successfully navigated through the murky waters of traumatic brain injury, through years of rehabilitation and adjustment. Instead of staying mired in anger, they took action: James Brady became the National Honorary Chairperson of the Brain Injury Association in 1989. And both he and his wife became leading advocates for gun control. Together, they saw their hard work pay off with the signing of the Brady Bill, which regulates the sale and use of guns.

A less famous but no less heroic tale comes from a woman whose teen-age son had come to HealthSouth RIOSA with a severe brain injury. The prognosis was dire; the distressed mother was told to accept what was, that her son would never recover. She refused to give up hope. Instead, she stayed with her son, by his bedside; she became an integral part of his rehabilitation "team." A year and a half later, he is living at home, coming in to the hospital only for group and speech therapy. As she told us, "All of us have to face reality. It's like there's this person, an adult. Then there's the accident; then another person emerges. You have to learn new ways of living. You have to cope with a new life. All of us need to cope with what's left. I have something to live for. My son is alive."

Believe in hope. Not false hope, but real hope. And channel the anger, the disappointment, and the pain into something stronger: change. You can make a difference.

CHAPTER FOUR

IN THE FIRST DEGREE: MILD HEAD INJURY

"It was the 'ding,' the sound in my head that started it all.
I was playing football, I never lost consciousness,
but I fell to the ground. I felt foggy, out of sorts, I couldn't
remember anything about the game. I never thought
I had a brain injury. I didn't get knocked out.
But something was wrong. Absolutely."

An 18-year-old HealthSouth outpatient
suffering from mild head injury

Joe is one of the best house painters around. But one particularly humid, hot day is getting to him. He can barely lift his arm; the smell of the paint is making him light-headed. He just wants to finish that last panel by the patio — almost done ... a scream! Joe falls off his ladder onto the grass. He's dazed, holding his head, and moaning. The homeowner, running outside as she hears Joe yell, is relieved that he is conscious. He keeps telling her he's fine, but his speech is slurred. He had taken a tough spill and she calls an ambulance, just in case. By the time it arrives 10 minutes later, Joe is sitting up. At the hospital, he's diagnosed as suffering from mild head injury. His CT scan shows that his brain is normal. After a few hours, he's discharged from the hospital, ready to go back to work.

But over the next few days, physical and psychological difficulties develop. Joe becomes irritable. He can't remember simple things. He's restless, and he simply can't work on the task at hand. It takes forever to paint even the porch of one house. Unfortunately, his clients don't appreciate this.

There's little sympathy. After all, they are paying Joe to paint their homes....

Fired from job after job, Joe becomes extremely depressed. He tries to get a job working as a painter for a large contractor, but he can only handle it for three weeks before he's fired once again. His depression spirals down, pushing his friends and his family further and further away. His wife starts to complain; Joe just isn't there anymore. He doesn't seem to care about the kids, and he gets so angry. Frankly, she's afraid.

Four months have now gone by. Joe's wife has left him, taking the kids. Joe is miserable. He has angry outbursts. There's only one thing that makes him feel better: alcohol. He starts to drink. He continues to drink. Soon, he does nothing but drink.

It isn't until a concerned friend gets him to enter an alcohol abuse program at a local hospital that Joe's problems are finally addressed. A neurologist on the hospital staff orders a series of neuropsychological tests, which reveal that Joe has persistent post-concussive syndrome (PPCS), a form that mild head injury may take. At last Joe will receive the brain injury rehabilitation treatment he so desperately needs.

THE "DING-A-LING ... ER"

It bears repeating: There are currently over 5.3 million people suffering from some form of traumatic brain injury and each year, over 2 million more people join them. That's one person every 15 seconds! Today, even with new, enforced safety regulations, including seat belt and helmet laws, and millions of government dollars appropriated to brain injury research, the number remains high. Unfortunately, the numbers may be higher still and simply not being recorded. Fewer and fewer people are going to emergency rooms or doctors' offices when they hit their heads; when people suffer mild head injuries, that ding, that bang, that ouch! that quickly passes, they might ignore it, especially if their dizziness, disorientation, or pain soon subsides.

These are the mild head injuries — from an aggressive tackle on the football field to a slip on the ice, from an accidental "ding" when a kitchen cabinet hits your head when opened to a coworker's door accidentally pushed open as you were about to enter.

Seventy-five percent of all brain injuries are these mild head injuries, categorized by:

- No loss of consciousness — or one so brief that it lasts less than 15 minutes
- A dazed, vacant stare right after the injury
- A normal neurological examination
- Delayed motor response to questions, such as "touch your nose"
- Disorientation and foggy memory
- Headaches, dizziness, or nausea
- Slurred speech
- A normal CT scan or MRI

Because the signs and symptoms of mild head injury are similar to other problems, it is often misdiagnosed. Like Joe, the house painter, people with a normal CT scan and no loss of consciousness may be sent on their way. In fact, 50% of those who suffer a mild head injury go back to work within two weeks. But one-third are unemployed three to six months after their accident — and 15%, like Joe, continue to suffer with depression, irritability, and headaches, symptoms which, collectively, are called persistent post-concussive syndrome (PPCS).

THE "MILD" TRIANGLE

Genuine symptoms of mild head injury that may result in PPCS are a combination of the physical, neurological, and psychological. It might be difficult for you to realize that your loved one is really in pain, especially when he looks and sounds just fine, but these symptoms are very real to him — and they may get worse if he does not receive the treatment he needs. Here's a brief summary of the three types of symptoms:

Triangle Side 1: A Physical Education

A headache or a feeling of dizziness after an accident may be a sign of mild head injury. They usually occur soon or right after the fall. A delayed onset suggests that something else is the cause of the problem. Dizziness may be the result of a change in position of the head; it can also be a vague sense of imbalance. Headaches can become excruciating — migraines combined with nausea, vomiting, and blurred vision. You may also feel constant pressure. Other physical symptoms include:

- Overall fatigue
- A sensitivity to light and noise
- Numbness or tingling in the hands and feet
- Ringing in the ears, or tinnitus

Triangle Side 2: Mind Your Mind

Memory loss is a critical factor in any brain injury —

HEADLINERS

A UNIQUE FEELING

The severity of psychological and emotional symptoms of mild head injury are influenced by a person's temperament and psychological makeup before the injury took place. We are all different, individuals, who react to life and its ups and downs in our own ways. Those who suffer a mild head injury are no exception: Was she an anxious person to begin with? Was he irritable and depressed? Did she suffer from insomnia?

A history of drug abuse and alcoholism can also substantially increase these symptoms — as well as possibly triggering the head injury in the first place!

---

and mild head injury is no exception. Your loved one might have difficulty remembering what you just said — or the name of someone he just met. She might forget her children's birthdays. He might forget what he went to buy at the grocery store. Other cognitive problems may include:

- Difficulty concentrating
- Increased distractibility
- Difficulty reading
- Inability to pay attention or solve problems

Cognitive problems usually show up quite clearly within the first month of an injury. But studies have found that these symptoms may, in a small group of patients, remain as long as two years after the accident. These symptoms may be subtle; they might not show up until a person is in a stressful situation or very distracted. You and your loved one might not, at first, associate them with the accident. The result? Reduced performance. An attorney might lose his edge in quickly reassessing trial strategies. She might find it hard to present her case in a logical, sequential manner. A secretary might begin to misfile documents—or forget important phone numbers.

Triangle Side 3: More than Feelings

Depression. It's the most common psychological problem after a mild head injury. In fact, studies have found that there might be a connection between the depression and the physical symptoms of dizziness, weakness, and fatigue. The depression may have come first, after the injury, triggering the physical symptoms. Other psychological symptoms include:

- Increased anxiety
- Mood swings
- Sleep disturbances
- Irritability
- Loss of libido

You and the other members of your family may be the best judges of these symptoms; you are better able to determine if your loved one is irritable or anxious, moody, or depressed.

MILD MANNERS

A mild head injury occurs during the same *acceleration-deceleration* action, the same basic mechanism that occurs in more serious injuries. The difference is one of degrees, based on speed, direction, and impact. But head injury, by its very definition, is an accident, a jolt from the blue. The sudden head movement created by the injury can stretch the nerve fibers, or axons, in the brain. Like a muscle or joint, they can become strained, resulting in only temporary symptoms. Most mild head injuries are a "strain," and people usually recover within three months. But sometimes these "strains" result in persistent problems with symptoms that come and go — and which can get worse as time goes by. The result? Persistent post-concussive syndrome (PPCS), which is usually a combination of physical and emotional problems.

Who suffers from PPCS? Who genuinely has symptoms of mild head injury? And who is fraught with anxiety, distress, and other psychological problems — and who is intentionally exaggerating symptoms? Deciding if it's really "all in your head" is one of the questions that has been the subject of lengthy debates among doctors and lawyers.

IT'S NOT JUST A GAME

It's a hot, humid night in America's suburbs. The local high school football team is playing a visiting team from another town. Everyone is at the game, cheering their team on as night settles in. The crickets vie with the roar of the crowd, the floodlights surrounding the grassy field go on. The star quarterback, "Bubba" Collins, goes out for the pass and is clobbered simultaneously from all sides.

He's down. He doesn't move as the other players pile off him. He stares vacantly ahead. The referee blows his whistle for time out; the crowd is silent. "Bubba! Bubba! Can you hear me?"

Bubba continues to stare straight ahead; he's conscious, but he's not with the crowd. The coach shouts: "Bubba, what city are we in? What was the last play?"

Nothing. But, finally, after a few minutes that seem like hours, Bubba gets to his feet. He has a headache and his reaction time seems slow. Yet by halftime Bubba is back on the field, a little shaky, but still ready to play. The crowd calls him a trooper; the coach slaps him on the back.

But Bubba is still dazed. He'd seen stars and they've only dimmed. Two weeks later, he was tackled again on the field. He had another concussion; this time, his performance on the field was affected. He began to do poorly in school; he couldn't remember dates. Bubba was seeing the result of multiple concussions, the symptoms that accumulate until they are severe enough to be noticed. With each tackle, his neurological symptoms increased. His first mild head injury had turned into something more serious. Like a boxer who's continually knocked out in the ring, Bubba had become "punch drunk," exhibiting symptoms of memory impairment, disorientation, clumsiness, and shakiness.

Bubba should never have gone back to the playing field. He had suffered a mild head injury and he needed to recuperate. He may have needed rehabilitation. But he seemed fine, if a little dazed. *He wanted to play.*

THE "SIDELINE EXAM"

If Bubba's coach had taken a few moments to do what we call the "sideline exam," perhaps the young star wouldn't have had a second concussion on top of the first; he would have received the treatment he needed. Here's the simple test. Like CPR, it's something every family member, every educator, every coworker and coach should know:

• *Reality check.* Is the injured person oriented and aware

of his surroundings? Bubba's coach should ask him who he is, where he is, the day and time, and if he understands the current situation.

• *The game of concentration.* Can the injured person focus on a specific question? Is his attention span still within normal ranges? Bubba's coach should ask him to do some quick and easy multiplication. He should ask him to name the months of the year — backwards.

• *Down Memory Lane.* Is the injured person's memory impaired? Bubba's coach should ask him to immediately repeat three objects and three numbers. Five minutes later, he should ask him again.

• *A stress test.* Do his thinking problems worsen with exercise? If Bubba could do five push-ups, five sit-ups, five knee bends, and a quick 40-yard sprint without his ability to think getting worse, he would have passed this portion of the "sideline exam." The coach should ask him to repeat the exercises to make sure nothing crops up that would have easily been missed if Bubba was sitting on the bench.

• *Neurologist for a minute.* How are the injured person's eyes? Does he seem to have a loss of perception? Is he weak? Bubba's trainer should check his pupils and his strength carefully.

In short, watch for signs of potential problems. Don't be so quick to let Bubba back in the game — no matter how loud the crowd is roaring. If all seems well after 15 minutes, you could let him back on the field, but keep performing the "sideline exam." Be alert to any changes that may occur five minutes, 15 minutes, several hours, and even several days later.

TIMING IS EVERYTHING

Like Joe, the house painter, or Bubba, hesitating when a mild head injury occurs can mean the loss of valuable time. The sooner a person enters a program, the better the results. They need to understand why they feel the way they do before they can start to work on their problems. Education is power. Many people become anxious and distressed because they don't know why they hurt. Early intervention can prevent the injury from becoming persistent post-concussive syndrome.

The exact figures aside, the main point to remember is that *time is of the essence in head injury*. Joe was in fact hospitalized after his fall from the ladder, but no one realized the extent of his brain injury. If someone had correctly diagnosed his continuing problems, and made sure he got

---

HEADLINERS

BY THE NUMBERS

- *Young people between the ages of 16 and 25 are more active and will suffer mild head injury from sports and at work.*
- *People over 65 are more prone to falls at home, resulting in mild head injury. A hint: Remove "throw rugs" from your parents' house. It decreases their chances of slipping.*
- *Alcohol intoxication plays a nasty role in brain injury because it predisposes people to act recklessly — especially behind the wheel of a car. Drinking and driving should never mix, but too often they do.*

HEADLINERS

MALINGERING: FACT OR FICTION?

Worse than the lack of quick detection is the fact that many doctors scoff off PPCS as malingering — a way for a "needy" victim to get attention or compensation. Still others claim, "It's all in his head." In reality, as study after study has shown, persistent post-concussive syndrome is likely to be a combination of both neurological and psychological problems. Incidentally, a few of the head-injured patients we have treated have been malingerers, particularly when lawsuits or workers' compensation is involved.

---

proper rehabilitation as soon as possible, Joe could have avoided much anguish and pain. Now, he not only has to be treated for the neurological damage his injury caused, but also for depression and alcoholism.

And Bubba could be going down the same dangerous and costly road.

But mild head injury is exactly that: mild. It doesn't have to develop into PPCS. Symptoms don't have to get worse. Just remember: Trust your instincts. Listen to your body and your mind. If things don't seem right, get it checked out — immediately. It might be a cliché, but it really is better to be safe than sorry.

To help you detect the symptoms of brain injury in yourself or a loved one, let's go on to diagnosis — and see how doctors become brain injury detectives.

CHAPTER FIVE

THE DOCTOR AS DETECTIVE

*"I thought my headaches were nothing but stress —
until my doctor insisted I go for neuropsychological
testing. I was nervous, but it was worth it. The mild
head injury had caused my outbursts —
and now I'm doing better. I'm calmer."*

An accountant who came to
HealthSouth on an outpatient basis

Ned, a prominent TV personality, hated the idea of turning 30. He knew that his looks and his health translated directly into success on the job. What Ned didn't know was that within a few short weeks, he'd be hoping to turn thirtysomething. It happened on a particularly sultry Los Angeles evening as he leaned against the railing of a second-floor apartment balcony, chatting with a woman he'd just met. Suddenly the railing gave way. Ned fell, struck his head on the concrete below and lost consciousness.

This is what his acute-care hospital report said:

"In the emergency room he presented with a Glasgow Coma Scale of 6. CT scan revealed large blood clots over the surface of the left brain and a smaller one over the right side. There was a large bruise involving the right parietal region. The patient underwent approximately 3 hours of brain surgery and remained comatose and poorly responsive for two weeks. He started to awaken with poorly localized responses, only withdrawing an arm or leg to painful stimuli. He did not produce speech, nor did he show any recognition of voice. He subsequently made rapid physical improvement, being able to ambulate and speak. However, he had significant problems with confusion and disorientation..."

No, this is not shorthand medical lingo that only doctors with 20 years of experience could understand. What this report clearly presents in one brief paragraph is a brain injury diagnosis. After you've read this chapter, you will understand the meaning of that diagnosis and others.

ONE, TWO, THREE, TESTING...

A study of patients undergoing brain injury testing found that they were particularly likely to have *emotional* distress if their injury had occurred more than six months before and they had not received any help. These patients were apt to be anxious, depressed, confused, and socially withdrawn. The fact is that the sooner rehabilitation starts, the sooner the recovery process can begin. But before you can set up a treatment program, you need at least a preliminary diagnosis. And that starts with some basic diagnostic tools:

1. CT SCAN. Computerized Axial Tomography (CAT for short) has pretty much taken over the job plain X-rays used to do, especially for suspected brain injuries. Although a CT scanner looks like something from a science-fiction movie, this large, donut-shaped machine is actually an X-ray camera that can take pictures of a person's brain in slices. Because it is able to photographically "peel away" layers of tissue, it can pinpoint problem areas, especially bruises and blood accumulation. A CT scan can help determine if surgery is needed — CT scans are an especially good tool for exploring open brain injury wounds. In fact, studies have found that CT scans have an almost 100% accuracy rate in identifying blood clots. But nerve damage, which can be extremely subtle, may not be picked up in initial CT scans. Blood that seeps slowly from damaged tissues beneath the skull (called *subdural hematomas*) can also go unnoticed. Unfortunately, that means that the seeping blood has a chance to accumulate and put undue pressure on the brain, which leads to more nerve damage. As you can see, more finely tuned diagnostic tools are needed. Luckily, such tools exist in today's world.

2. MRI stands for Magnetic Resonance Imaging. Now for what it means: combining physics and computer technology, MRIs are able to pinpoint problems that would never be seen on a CT scan. Like a highly evolved detector, an MRI uses radio frequencies and a magnet to chart the energy in the brain; it then converts them into computerized, highly detailed pictures of the brain. MRIs can display both focal and diffuse nerve damage.

But when it comes to minor brain injuries that cause subtle cognitive damage, even the sophistication of an MRI might not be enough...

3. PET Scan. A PET (Positron Emission Tomography) scan creates an actual map of the patient's brain. A tagged radioactive liquid is injected; as the liquid seeps throughout the brain, its movements are tracked and an individual portrait is created. PET scans have been found to show minor brain abnormalities that are not picked up by an MRI.

4. EEG. In an electroencephalogram (EEG), electrodes attached to the scalp measure the electrical activity (waves) in the brain and show the results, either on graph paper or on a display screen. If someone has a moderate or severe head injury, chances are it will show up as an abnormal brain wave pattern or in an irregular brain wave speed.

5. Evoked Potentials. These are relatives of the EEG. Rather than passively measuring electrical activity, evoked potentials measure the brain's ability to respond to specific visual, auditory, and sensory stimuli. In selected patients, they may help determine if the sensory pathways in the brain are damaged.

Other diagnostic tools you might hear mentioned include intracranial pressure monitoring, cerebral blood flow measurement, and measurements of cerebral metabolism.

THE ART OF PREDICTION

In addition to the tools created by modern technology, there are other useful predictors of outcome that have evolved through much research and scientific study. These low-tech predictors count on experienced doctors' abilities to analyze and diagnose a head injury. The way the patient feels, reacts, and functions are key components in making a diagnosis. In medical detective work, the patient himself provides the most important clues of all.

Here's a brief description of these other tools that are used in rehabilitation hospitals nationwide:

Tool #1: The Glasgow Coma Scale

Imagine a technique so simple that everyone, from the most highly trained neurologist to the newest nurse in the emergency ward, could use it to determine the severity of injury within those first crucial hours. This does in fact exist. It's the Glasgow Coma Scale, a universal system that rates the severity of a person's injury by his ability to open his eyes, move, and speak. The more severe the injury, the lower his performance, and the lower the number he is assigned. A very low number suggests very serious injury, and little likelihood of total recovery.

Here's a twist: Severe injury doesn't always imply deep unconsciousness.

It all has to do with the number on the scale, As far as gross observable changes go, the Glasgow Coma Scale works so well that it has only a 3% disagreement rate.

Here's what the scale looks like:

GLASGOW COMA SCALE

Eye opening
Spontaneously 4
To speech 3
To pain 2
None 1

Best motor response
Obeys commands 6
Moves within the general locale 5
Withdraws 4
Abnormal muscle bending and flexing 3
Involuntary muscle straightening and extending 2
None 1

Verbal response

Is oriented 5
Confused conversation 4
Inappropriate words 3
Incomprehensible sounds 2
None..1

But as good a common denominator as it is, the Glasgow Coma Scale does have its limitations. Yes, it does its job of predicting outcome and certainly helps determine whether someone will live or die. It gives a broad measure of how well someone will recover. But it does not predict whether someone will live independently or be able to work competently, even when they have a good recovery.

Other predictors of outcome are needed.

Tool #2: Post-Traumatic Amnesia (PTA)

As you can probably guess, this predictor has to do with memory. In fact, it's a useful guide to determine cognitive outcome within the first year.

Here's how it *doesn't* work:

When a brain-injured patient wakes up from being unconscious, he doesn't sit upright and cheerfully ask for the person he loves. Nor does he ask for some good, hot food, as actors are prone to do on primetime soaps.

Here's how it *does* work:

Waking up is an extremely gradual process, and the part of the conscious mind that takes the *longest* to recover is memory. The loss of remembering day-to-day events after injury is so prevalent, in fact, that it has a name: *Post-Traumatic Amnesia.*

PTA is categorized from the moment of the accident to the time when a patient becomes lucid, remembering day-to-day events in a continuous memory. The longer the memory loss after the accident, the more serious the injury — and the less the chances for a good recovery.

In the interim, before their memory clicks in, brain-injured patients may not understand where they are or even *who* they are. Some patients become extremely agitated and cannot be comforted. When their memory comes back, they usually have little or no recollection of their hours, days, or months of post-traumatic amnesia time.

As a rule, a patient who has PTA for less than one hour is diagnosed as having a mild head injury. One to 24 hours translates into moderate head injury. Anything longer than 24 hours is considered severe. This is an important reality for families to face, because they usually feel absolutely joyous that their loved one awakens from a coma after "only" four days. *But* if both the Glasgow Coma Scale and PTA point to severe head injury, the patient will most likely have long-term cognitive and behavioral deficits.

PTA as a predictor tool is not absolute. It's difficult to pinpoint its time line exactly. Not only is the patient confused, but family members or significant others are usually too overwhelmed to recall accurately when their loved ones begin to remember. Then, too, as a patient regains consciousness, he'll be inconsistent, remembering the time one day but not the next, recalling your name at five o'clock but not at six. This makes it hard to use the PTA as a predictor of outcome. Thus other tests are still needed.

Tool #3: The Rancho Los Amigos Scale of Cognitive Functioning

Developed at California's Rancho Los Amigos Hospital, this scale is divided into eight stages with a gradual progression from deep coma to appropriate behavior and cognitive functioning. It is not really a predictor of outcome, but, rather, a tool to describe the person.

Why use the Rancho Los Amigos Scale? It's a quick, handy, universal shorthand to diagnose and communicate a patient's level of functioning. It also can be used to guide and develop individual rehabilitation programs. Here's a brief description of its eight stages:

Level I: No Response. The patient is unconscious. He appears to be sleeping. He does not respond to any stimuli presented to him. This comatose state can last for seconds, minutes, hours, days, weeks, or even months.

Level II: Generalized Response. Here, the patient will react, but inconsistently and without purpose. His response, often a gross body movement or a garbled vocalization, is usually the same, regardless of what Glasgow stimulus is used. But his first response is activated, more times than not, from deep pain.

Level III: Localized Response. The patient is improving. He will react more specifically to different stimuli, but his response will be inconsistent. For example, he may occasionally turn his head in the direction of a speaker's voice. He may have a vague awareness of his body. He may inconsistently follow simple commands such as "close your eyes" or "squeeze my hand."

Level IV: Confused-Agitated. The patient has become very active, but he is not yet able to understand what's going on. His behavior might become bizarre; he might cry out or try to remove his feeding tube. He may be hostile and unco-operative, but he is not acting out of malice. It's a reaction to his overwhelming confusion.

Level V: Confused-Inappropriate. The patient has become less agitated; he will respond to simple commands in a more consistent manner. But if the commands are more complex, he gets confused and gives random, incorrect responses. He may become agitated if he is in a noisy or "busy" environment. He will not take the initiative. He will respond best to his body's aches and pains, to his own comfort, and to close family members. His memory is severely impaired, and he is unable to learn new information. At this level, he is in danger of "wandering off" the ward.

Level VI: Confused-Appropriate. Things are looking up. The patient is motivated, but still depends on others to lead the way toward his goals. His reactions will be more appropriate. If he is uncomfortable he will complain. He is beginning to recognize therapy staff members, and is much more aware of himself and his family. He can easily follow simple directions. His memory of the past has improved greatly, but his memory of recent events is still impaired.

Level VII: Automatic-Appropriate. The patient seems to act appropriately in the hospital and at home. He is now ori-ented to person, place, and time in these settings. All seems well, but things are still not completely right. He may go through his daily routines automatically. Although he can dress, wash, and feed himself independently, he needs supervision to ensure his safety. His judgment and problem-solving skills are still impaired, and he cannot make realistic plans for his future.

Level VIII: Purposeful and Appropriate. At last! The patient can integrate the past with recent events. He is independent and functional in society. However, he may have subtle difficulties with reasoning, judgment, and processing information, especially in high stress, unusual, or emergency situations. He may be actively involved in a vocational rehabilitation program, learning a new way to live in his new world.

This hierarchy of levels looks simple and straightforward. But in real life, not every brain-injured survivor moves smoothly through each level. A patient may move from Level II to Level IV and never demonstrate any true Level III behaviors. Or, a patient may reach Level III and never progress beyond that point. Even if your loved one reaches Level VIII, it won't necessarily mean he is exactly as he once was. As mentioned earlier, he will most likely be changed — in ways that are subtle or not so subtle. To determine these "finely tuned" changes, medical professionals must turn to other means...

Tool #4: Neuropsychological Testing

Written questionnaires. Mazes. Blocks. Storybooks. These are some of the tools of the neuropsychological testing trade. Varied and carefully plotted, these tests can help determine within 4 to 10 hours what the previous diagnostic techniques may not:

HEADLINERS

YOU MUST REMEMBER THIS

We know families that keep trying and trying to get their brain-injured loved one to remember the accident that started it all. They'll coach their loved one as if the World Series were at stake, or at least the college boards. But in fact, the majority of brain-injured survivors never remember their accident. This has nothing whatsoever to do with their ability to recover. Call it ironic. Call it fascinating. But also call it normal.

- *Behavioral problems*, such as the capacity for violent outbursts or immature behavior
- *Emotional problems*, such as depression, anxiety, or distress
- *Cognitive problems*, such as sequencing difficulties or attention deficits

These tests can also help a rehabilitation team separate those dysfunctions caused by accident-related neurological damage from those with a psychological base. For example, memory complaints might be the result of temporal lobe damage and difficulty sustaining attention, or an emotional response to overwhelming stress and depression. Anxiety and depression can make it difficult to concentrate and attend to tasks. A person who's nervous tends to be forgetful.

Neuropsychological testing can also help identify a patient's primary problem and isolate it from any secondary problems it might have caused. Another example: Let's say a brain-injured person has trouble both comprehending what he reads and following instructions. However, tests performed by the rehabilitation team may show that these are only secondary problems caused by a primary problem: inability to pay attention. Tackle the attention deficit, and chances are the patient's comprehension and ability to follow directions will improve. Without outside distraction or with repetition he may be able to concentrate on what he's reading — and enjoy it more. Without the benefit of test results as a guide, a rehabilitation therapist might try everything in the book to improve a patient's reading comprehension — to no avail. Until the patient improves his attention skills, the other problems may never go away. Some of the neuropsychological tests include:

• *Serial addition test.* In this test the patient is asked to listen to numbers and add them together sequentially For example, he will hear 3 plus 5 and state "8." Then he will hear the number 5 and should respond "13." This is a sensitive test of memory skills.

• *Tactual performance test.* Here, the patient is blindfolded and seated at a table holding a board and 10 wooden blocks. He must replace all the blocks without looking, using first his dominant hand, then his nondominant hand. He's then instructed to take off his blindfold and draw the board and the blocks from memory.

Motor skills, problem solving, spatial and tactile memory, and learning ability can all be analyzed with this one simple test.

• *Finger tapping test.* Using a mechanical counter or a metronome, the patient taps in rhythm as rapidly as possible for 10 seconds, using both his dominant and nondominant hands. This test will tell a rehabilitation team if a patient has problems with motor speed.

• *The MMPI-2* (The Minnesota Multiphasic Personality Inventory - Revised). This 60 to 90 minute questionnaire is used in all aspects of psychological testing to determine how well a person can function in society; it helps define a person's personality, pinpointing any possible mental disorders as well as inappropriate behaviors. It is given to brain injury patients and their family members to determine how well everyone functions as a family unit, how capable a family is to help the brain-injured person, and whether family members themselves have any psychological problems that might have predisposed the patient to injury.

There's a real need for neuropsychological testing; it's an excellent tool that will tell you the specific cognitive and behavioral skills that need work. The tests have a 74% to 90% accuracy rate, but proper interpretation is crucial: They are only as good as the person interpreting them. A sensitive clinician must determine whether a patient's...

- Anxiety is an ongoing concern or simply pre-testing jitters.
- Behavioral problems were in place well before the injury.
- Primary and secondary problems are hidden by the unique, highly focused, one-on-one testing environment.

A patient might be at his best in the testing room, but only because he's the focus of one person's complete attention for hours.

Test results can also pinpoint secondary psychological problems. Immaturity, selfishness, rudeness, and depression can all come out not only during the testing procedure, but during break-time conversation.

Tool #5: Pre-injury Characteristics

Research has suggested that brain injury may not always strike entirely at random. Learning-disabled children, impulsive and aggressive young adults, alcohol- and drug-abusing adolescents — all are predisposed to injury. In fact, one particular study of brain-injured patients with a prehistory of drug abuse discovered that they had twice as many behavioral problems as patients who had never abused drugs. The behavioral problems didn't surface until late in the recovery process, frustrating family members and hospital staff alike.

The family circle also plays a role. Families with a brain-injured member have been found to have more depression, more instability, and more social disadvantages than other families.

Here are several pre-injury traits that assist a person's recovery:

• *A "fighter" personality.* Someone who had been strong before her accident, who was patient, who was motivated and achievement-oriented, stands a better chance of regaining these traits and getting through the rehabilitation process with success.

• *Youth.* Studies have found that fewer children die from head injuries than their adult counterparts. In fact, the younger the person, the better the chances of successful rehabilitation, (The reasons may involve the flexibility or "plasticity" of a child's brain, which we'll discuss later.)

• *Intelligence.* The smarter the person, the more likely he will benefit from rehabilitation techniques.

• *Self-control.* If a brain-injured person has been able to retain (or re-master) his self-control, he'll also be better able to control inappropriate behavior and impulsiveness, possibly re-entering the community much sooner than his out-of-control, undisciplined counterpart.

• *Strong family ties.* The more love, support, and encouragement the patient feels from his family, the more it will help his rehabilitation — and his future care. In fact, the role of the family is so crucial an issue in brain injury rehabilitation that we give the subject its own chapter.

• *Similarity of pre-injury career skills and post-injury skills.* If a brain-injured person had a fairly uncomplicated job, he'll probably have an easier time re-entering the job market than someone who is, say, a lawyer, whose organizational and memory problems may prevent him from exercising his profession.

• *Good coping skills.* Someone who knew how to relax and handle stress before her injury will cope better with the stress and trauma associated with brain injury.

• *Solid financial support.* It's a fact of life: Rehabilitation

---

HEADLINERS

Here is a situation that took place between a brain-injured boy, overwhelmed by his central nervous system problems, and his nurse one morning at HealthSouth RIOSA:

The nurse had repeatedly asked him to get out of bed and brush his teeth. The boy smiled at her and, as if to rise, pushed his blanket away with one hand. But his other hand was raised in a fist; he was shaking his hand while he was smiling. "Look out, because I'm going to have to hit you hard." The nurse paused and gently said, 'This is hard on you, Tommy, isn't it?" The boy, relieved that she understood, nodded. "Yes!"

---

can be expensive. In order to receive the best possible care, patients need either good financial resources or adequate health insurance. Unfortunately, many brain injury patients don't get all the help they need because they don't have adequate coverage — and they don't know where to turn. Good rehabilitation hospitals have case managers or social workers to help families find the resources they need, either through government funding or negotiating with their insurance carriers.

• *Deficit awareness.* More than anything else, a brain-injured patient must become aware of his problems. Even the most reputable and sophisticated rehabilitation program will not work as well if a person is unaware of his deficits. Deficit-awareness is crucial. A person must ultimately recognize his new limitations if he's to actively participate and return to his community.

As time marches on, these pre-injury characteristics become more and more important as diagnostic tools. A patient's personality, his lifestyle, his coping skills, his home or hospital environment — all these play a major role in predicting ultimate success.

Before we close the file on this particular piece of detective work, it's important to remember that predictions may be wrong. Diagnostic tools, research, and scientific studies are the best we have, but we cannot tell which of the billions of brain cells are dead — and which are merely damaged. It is difficult, at first, to tell if a person will have some spon-

---

HEADLINERS

Some questions we use at HealthSouth RIOSA call for the patients to rate themselves so that we can see what they perceive they can do — and what their reality really is. For example:

How much of a problem do I have in...

... preparing my own meals?

... dressing myself?

... remembering names of people I see often?

... driving a car if I have to?

... controlling crying?

... recognizing when something I say or do has upset someone else?

... controlling my temper when something upsets me?

---

taneous recovery We cannot tell early on with certainty which patient will plateau and never get beyond, say, Rancho Los Amigos Level V. However, most patients experience a large part of their recovery the first year; we also know that improvement can continue for years.

• *Recovery takes time.* The symptoms that appear after a brain injury can linger for a long while. They can even create more symptoms with a life of their own. To cope with this confusing time, you should understand what the possible symptoms are and why they may exist in your brain-injured loved one. Let's go on to these symptoms now.

CHAPTER SIX

PHYSICAL SYMPTOMS OF BRAIN INJURY

"I used to jog four miles a day to stay in shape.
Now I get to have my own personal trainer.
I have a physical therapist who works on
my legs... They won't move."

A former high school star at
HealthSouth RIOSA

Susan loved to feel the wind in her hair. In fact, that was one of the main reasons she loved to ride her bicycle. Eight years ago, when the city had had a transportation strike, getting to and from work became everyone's biggest problem. Susan got out her old rusty three-speeder. Within the first half-mile down the avenue, she'd regained her balance, her speed, and her love for bike riding.

The years went by. The strike was long over, but Susan continued to ride her bike wherever she went. She began to take weekend biking trips in the country. Some of the people she met on her trips wore helmets, but Susan thought that was being overly cautious. She referred to the helmets as "the new Yuppie toy."

Unfortunately, Susan didn't have the last laugh. On her ride out of the city one Friday night, she hit a pothole that she never even saw. She was flung over the handlebars, and hit her head on the concrete street.

By the time the ambulance brought her to the nearest hospital, Susan had already regained consciousness. But she was confused; she couldn't remember what had happened.

A CT scan showed some bruising in her frontal and temporal lobes and a large blood clot in her brain. The brain had swelled, and intracranial pressure was building. Susan was rushed into surgery. After four hours on the operating table, she was put in intensive care and watched around the clock, receiving medication to reduce the swelling further and to prevent seizures. Eventually she was referred to a rehabilitation hospital.

Susan was alive and awake; she remembered who and where she was. Her parents were grateful that they had their daughter back. Her friends and coworkers were relieved. None of them — not even Susan herself — knew how close she had come to death, not because of her initial fall, but because of the secondary physical problems the brain injury caused.

Before being tested for any neurological or psychological problems, before tackling any cognitive retraining, a brain-injured person literally has to fight for her life. One life-threatening result of her injury may be hematoma.

HEMATOMA

When the brain is bruised, it may bleed. The more it bleeds, the more it will swell, and the larger the accumulation of blood. The act of bleeding is called *hemorrhage* and the collection of blood is called a *hematoma*. Now, when this pool of blood actually fills up within the brain, it's known as an *intracerebral hematoma*. When the blood is collecting between the brain and the dura (which, as described in Chapter One, is a durable membrane that covers the brain), it's called a *subdural hematoma*.

It might not be easy to stop a bleeding hand or leg, but at least the bleeding is visible. When the brain bleeds, it's all internal — nothing can be seen. And, as you saw in Chapter Five, even the most sophisticated diagnostic tools don't always pick up a deadly bruise.

But there's more: *The more the brain is damaged, the greater the risk of secondary swelling and bleeding.*

Unfortunately, as we explained earlier, swelling and bleeding go hand in hand to create a dangerous buildup of pressure, which can damage even more brain cells than the initial head injury did.

What happens to this swollen brain? Unless the intracranial pressure is relieved by medication or surgery, the ever-expanding brain will find space only by pushing and squeezing down on the brainstem, the all-important area of the brain that regulates vital functions, from heartbeat to breathing.

Think of it: The heartbeat slows. The breath is barely audible. Biochemical and mechanical functions of the brain go haywire, leading to widespread damage throughout the entire body. The brain's blood flow trickles down to nothing. The brain no longer receives the bloodstream's life-giving oxygen, resulting in *hypoxia*. Ultimately, more brain cells die, causing brain tissue death.

Susan was lucky. She was injured in a large city, where she was taken to a hospital quickly and received the care she needed. Her brain swelling (or edema) was brought down; damage was minimal. After rehabilitation, she returned to her city life and her job as before — with one crucial difference. She got herself the best bike helmet money could buy.

PHYSICAL EDUCATION

Secondary medical problems that can result from a brain injury are only part of the story. The physical symptoms or deficits that the injury causes tell another tale. Let's examine some of these symptoms now.

Seizures

In ancient times, epilepsy was considered a curse from the gods — for understandable reasons. When epilepsy occurs as a result of brain injury it can occasionally cause further injury. Any seizure starts with a burst of abnormal electrical activity somewhere in the brain. Seizures come in several different types:

Generalized or grand mal seizures are full-blown, involving widespread muscle contractions, rapid body movements, loss of bladder and bowel control, irregular breathing, and loss of consciousness. There is usually no warning. However, some patients do know when they are going to have a seizure; we call this feeling an aura. A common aura is a full feeling in the pit of the stomach that moves up toward the mouth.

Partial or focal seizures are a more subtle variety. Here, the brain-injured person merely has a total lapse of concentration. She might lose the thread of what she was doing, or stop talking in midsentence, or perform a repetitive task such as picking at her clothes. Partial seizures, which frequently arise from the temporal lobe, may be difficult to diagnose. A common form is called complex partial seizures. Focal seizures may involve jerking movements of only one arm or leg, without loss of consciousness.

Seizures occur in 35% of patients with open head

injuries, Although most seizures occur within the first week after an injury, the first one may not occur until one to two years following the brain injury Regardless of the time lag, the technical term for seizure following a brain injury is post-traumatic epilepsy.

Seizures are unpredictable. A patient may not be considered free of symptoms until two or three seizure-free years have passed. Even then, there is a small chance that another seizure will occur down the road. Epilepsy needs to be carefully monitored by a physician who is familiar with the correct use of antiseizure medication.

The good news is that only 1% of closed head injury patients develop seizures. Therefore, most of these patients do not need to be placed on medication.

Loss of Motor Control and Coordination

A brain-injured survivor in a wheelchair, learning to use it on different terrains... A right-handed man with *hemiplegia* (paralysis of either the right or left side of the body), learning to write with his left hand... A woman with *ataxia*, an awkward, unbalanced, and uncoordinated way of walking... A former athlete whose muscle strength and endurance is weakened, relearning to lift weights... A woman who appears frozen in time, her joints rigid and set in a beckoning pose... An adult man lying curled up in a fetal position, immobile... A knitter who can no longer hold her knitting needles, whose fingers have lost their agility and dexterity... A man whose motions are quick and brisk, quivering in spasticity... Physical impairments such as these are much easier to detect than cognitive or behavioral deficits, because they involve the parts of the brain that control what we can observe at a glance: body movement, muscle tone, and balance.

You may recall reading or hearing that the left side of the brain controls the right side of the body, and vice versa. A brain injury survivor with a blood clot or contusion on one side of the brain may have paralysis of the opposite side of the body; this is called hemiparesis or hemiplegia. Paralysis is commonly more severe in the arm than in the leg. As time passes, it's possible that the person will regain the ability to move his arm, but still won't be able to manage finely coordinated movements such as buttoning a shirt or manipulating coins. Therapists will help him work on increasing his strength and compensating for those lost muscle functions.

Walking difficulty, called *ataxia*, may respond to physical therapy and medications, but is often very difficult to treat. It's frustrating when the person has enough physical strength to walk, but lacks the necessary sense of balance. Such a person usually needs to adapt to using a wheelchair.

Spasticity, which is abnormally increased muscle tone frequently seen in paralyzed arms and legs, interferes with movement and can also be painful. It frequently improves in response to changes in position and also to stretching exercises. (A stretching routine, incidentally, is very important for almost all brain injury survivors).

Medications, including Lioresal® (baclofen), Zanaflex® (tizanidine), Dantrium® (dantrolene sodium), and Valium® (diazepam), can be useful in treating spasticity. However, these medications are a mixed blessing because they may also cause weakness and sedation. If a patient needs all his available muscle tone in order to walk, the medication that relieves his spasticity may actually prevent him from walking. Thus, the doctor who prescribes the medication must carefully consider the relative weight of benefits versus side effects.

New Hope for Spasticity

For many brain-injured survivors, medication and exercise don't spell enough relief from painful spasticity. Fortunately, today's physicians have some amazing things in their bag of tricks.

You still should throw that possibly contaminated can away, but, today, an old foe and a new friend, botulinum toxin (Botox®) can be injected safely into individual muscles of the arm or leg. This highly diluted toxin can be used to safely weaken overactive muscles, allowing spastic clenched fingers to open, decreasing pain and improving hygiene. Because Botox® is limited by the amount that can be injected at one time, it works best in the smaller muscles of the arms.

The larger muscles of the legs need much more Botox® than can be effectively injected in order to work. Here, the answer is intrathecal baclofen (ITB).

In pill form, baclofen can cause dizziness and drowsiness when taken in the higher doses needed for large muscle groups. In addition, it is not all that effective in the treatment of brain spasticity. A small titanium pump, made by the Medtronic Corporation, can overcome this problem by intrathecal administration, which places tiny amounts of baclofen directly in the cerebrospinal fluid. The pump is about the size of a hockey puck and fits comfortably under the skin. Even better, the rate at which it delivers the baclofen can be adjusted as often as necessary by a doctor; all that's needed is a computer and a wand that is placed over the skin. For some patients this procedure can produce a dramatic reduction in spasticity and pain.

Talk with your doctor or rehabilitation team to see if you are good candidate for either Botox® or ITB. (A simple outpatient procedure can determine if ITB is right for you.)

Sensory Problems

Our sensory perceptions are a product of both cognitive and physical abilities. We need to have the capability to understand, analyze, and remember in order to recognize and process what we see, hear, touch, taste, and smell. But we also need the ability to sense something in the first place. We need to *physically* see, hear, touch, taste, or smell. Unfortunately, this physical ability may be lost with brain injury. Damage to the occipital lobe can cause blindness. Sometimes *diplopia,* or double vision, occurs as a result of cranial nerve damage or muscle imbalance. The visual fields can become constricted due to injury within the visual pathways to the higher-functioning portions of the brain.

Sensitivity in the mouth can change as a result of brain injury. Hot foods can seem so hot they can't be swallowed. Cold foods can seem much too frigid. And sometimes taste is totally lost, as well as the ability to hear sounds or feel objects.

Head injury frequently damages the nerves that carry the sense of smell: The person may be left with a faulty "sniffer" or none at all. Unfortunately, this type of damage rarely improves with time, since it stems from permanent destruction of the cells that respond to smells.

Sometimes the person recovering from a brain injury is perfectly capable of moving his arm or leg, but has a severe disability because he can no longer keep track of where it is in space: He has suffered *proprioception* damage. To appreciate the function of proprioception, close your eyes and then touch the tip of your nose. You knew just how to move your arm and hand, didn't you? That's because your proprioception was intact. To rehabilitation professionals, patients with proprioception difficulties present a major challenge.

Speaking and Swallowing Disorders

A person doesn't normally give her mouth too much thought, unless she's brushing her teeth, for instance, or putting on lipstick. But her oral muscle function may become severely limited in brain injury. She may have a hard time articulating the words she wants to say, because the muscles needed to produce speech have become weak or have lost their coordination. This condition, called *dysarthria*, may cause her speech to be extremely slurred, or slower or quieter than normal, making it hard for others to understand her. A person whose brain injury has damaged her ability to chew and swallow efficiently is said to have *dysphagia*. If the dysphagia is so severe that it results in malnutrition, or causes her to have a chronic problem with food falling into her airway, she may need to receive all her nutrition through a feeding tube.

Fatigue and Headaches

Fatigue and headaches affect nearly everyone at one time or another. Unfortunately, it's not simply a matter of "take two aspirin and call me in the morning" when brain injury is involved. Fatigue and head pain can interfere with rehabilitation, requiring breaks that will slow down the process and possibly create future problems.

It's important not to exercise to the point of fatigue and to devise a realistic schedule that includes rest periods. Inadequate rest can lead to increased agitation, behavior difficulties, and decreased attention.

Headaches are common following mild head injury, but do not signify new or increasing brain injury.

Most headaches can be successfully treated with the same medications that are used for migraine headaches.

Bladder and Bowel Incontinence

No, this doesn't just happen in old age. Loss of bladder and bowel control is a very real and very unnerving physical disability. It's also tied into cognitive awareness. Remember when you toilet-trained your child? It took time, patience, and self-knowledge. All this can fall apart when a person sustains a brain injury. The brain-injured survivor may have difficulty urinating, requiring intermittent catheterization (placing a tube in the bladder). Or she may suffer a loss of bladder control (incontinence). Incontinence can be treated by offering her the opportunity to go to the bathroom every two hours. Occasionally formal bladder tests (urodynamics) are needed to identify the problem clearly. Most people with bladder trouble can be kept dry through medication, catheterization, and timed voiding. Likewise, timed bowel programs can prevent embarrassing mishaps. Constipation frequently responds to increasing intakes of fluid, fiber, and fruit. Bowel stimulants,

---

HEADLINERS

ALCOHOL AND BRAIN INJURY DON'T MIX

A study of 102 brain injury survivors admitted to a trauma center found that those who had been under the influence of alcohol at the time of admission were:

- *More agitated for a long period of time*
- *Discharged with lower cognitive abilities*
- *More neurologically and behaviorally affected by their injury*
- *More apt to ultimately die at a young age*

In addition, people who have been brain-injured have a lowered tolerance for alcohol. Depression, physical limitations, and the lack of access to quality long-term care makes many brain injury survivors turn to alcohol as a way to cope with their problems. Of course, alcohol ultimately makes their problems even worse.

---

stool softeners, and bulking agents can relieve constipation for most people.

As difficult as some of these physical impairments seem, they are actually the easiest ones to accept and rehabilitate. In fact, a study by Dr. Yehuda Ben-Yishay found that over 80% of brain-injured patients had an excellent physical recovery by the end of one year. The more lasting problems came from cognitive and behavioral deficit. These were the ones that determined the patients' ultimate social and personal adjustments — or, in other words, their ability to function once again in society

It's easier to cope with someone in a wheelchair than someone who hurls abuse at every turn. It's also more accepted. The physically handicapped are finally getting the recognition they need and deserve, from access ramps to Braille-numbered elevators, from closed captions to convenient parking spaces.

Unfortunately brain injury also causes invisible symptoms. Perhaps you sat next to one of the "walking wounded" when you rode the train to work this morning. Or, closer to home, perhaps your brain-injured husband just doesn't laugh the way he used to in that carefree way that made you fall in love with him. Worse yet, what if he doesn't remember getting married to you — or even what your name is?

An employer typically has less patience than a spouse or family member for these "walking wounded" brain injury survivors. A C.E.O. will proudly cut the ribbon to inaugurate the company's new offices built with access ramps for the handicapped. He'll have his picture taken with his first employee in a wheelchair. But he'll find it hard to justify paying someone who throws typewriters against the wall, can't meet deadlines, and refuses to get along with coworkers.

In short, physical problems are difficult, but cognitive and behavioral deficits can be an even greater handicap. Learning what the cognitive and behavioral symptoms are will help you cope and help the person you love get better. Let's move on to examine these "invisible," yet very noticeable, effects of brain injury.

CHAPTER SEVEN

COGNITIVE SYMPTOMS OF BRAIN INJURY

"I think, therefore I am."
Rene Descartes

Lorraine had always been a topnotch secretary. In fact, her firm voted her Secretary of the Year six years in a row. But then Lorraine was in an accident — a car driven by a drunk driver smashed into her car's rear end. She lost consciousness for almost half an hour. When she came to in the emergency room, she was confused. She couldn't remember what had happened. The diagnosis? Lorraine had a closed head injury with damage to her frontal and temporal lobes. Later, after three weeks at an acute-care hospital, she was admitted to a rehabilitation hospital.

While Lorraine was recuperating, everyone from work sent flowers. Her boss visited her once a week; her friends called at least once every other day. Within a month, Lorraine appeared to have regained her memory. She progressed rapidly, and after six months she was speaking and walking on her own. She could read, attend to her daily hygiene, and, all in all, seemed independent and ready to get on with her life.

The day Lorraine returned to the office, the entire staff threw her a party. There were strawberries and champagne, a three-layered cake, and a leather attaché case as a gift. Lorraine was exhilarated. She'd never felt happier in her life; she'd never appreciated life more. She couldn't wait to get back to her desk and begin working again.

That first week, all went well. Lorraine was the embodiment of confidence. She came into her boss's office, steno pad in hand, efficient and raring to go every time her boss buzzed. Lorraine told the boss not to worry — she would handle that MacGregor account herself. She would also do some research into that company they were thinking of buying. Lorraine said she planned on staying late the next few days so that she could refile all the notes on that Smith & Stein debacle.

But two weeks went by and Lorraine's boss had only signed about four letters. She had yet to see the research on the new firm, and MacGregor was calling her twice a day now about his account. She didn't know what to do. She cared about Lorraine, but the work wasn't getting done.

Something had to be done. One evening, after Lorraine had bid her good night, the boss sat down at Lorraine's desk. She had never snooped before, but she had to see for herself what was going on.

She was shocked. Lorraine's steno pads were filled with pencil sketches of flowers and random words in flowing script. Work to be filed was stashed away in a drawer. The files themselves were a mess, unalphabetized and overflowing. There were no notations on MacGregor, the new firm, or anything else for that matter. Just dirty coffee cups, drawings, and empty Cheetos bags...

When the boss confronted her the next day, Lorraine was aghast. She couldn't understand what the problem was. She had said she'd handle the MacGregor account, she just needed a little time. She would be happy to type up some letters, but she had misplaced her steno pad. And as far as the new firm was concerned, she had been about to make some calls when she was buzzed to come in. Why was her boss giving her such a hard time?

Clearly something was wrong. Lorraine was defensive. Both she and her boss knew she wasn't doing her work, but neither one knew why. They hadn't a clue. Her boss had no choice but to let her go. She gave Lorraine a decent severance package, but Lorraine was heartsick. She just needed time, that's all. She shouldn't have been fired; there wasn't enough cause. She tried to rally her coworkers against her boss; she wanted to sue the firm.

It all came to naught, however, because the Secretary of the Year could no longer handle the responsibilities of the job. Unfortunately, it had nothing to do with a sudden "mental breakdown." It had everything to do with Lorraine's brain injury seven months before.

Lorraine's story is only one out of thousands of incidents that occur each year. More than anything else, cognitive deficits mean a change of life.

KNOWLEDGE IS POWER

Cognitive meant "to know" in ancient Greek. Today, it means our intellectual, information-processing abilities. Performance, attention, organization, planning, memory, flexibility, perception, and sensitivity all come under the cognitive umbrella. Unfortunately, these intellectual lobes, which, as we have seen, usually get the thrust of a fall, an accident, or a traumatic assault.

Knowledge is power, and the root of its power is understanding. Before you can cope with a loved one's cognitive deficits, you must understand what they are. Before you can help a loved one regain his cognitive abilities, you have to know what is possible and what is not. Based on the classifications delineated by neuropsychologist George P. Prigatano, here are some aspects of cognition that may be faulty in a cognitively disabled person:

Mindset #1: Attention and Concentration

A driver doesn't see the light change from red to green at an intersection. A student is too busy listening to the "boom box" radio outside his classroom window to finish writing an essay on a test. A guest at a party stops in midsentence and abruptly begins talking about something else. These are all examples of attention and concentration deficits that may be daily occurrences for the brain injured.

Think of it: Without the ability to pay attention, a person can't work productively or even stay involved in a conversation in a social setting. In fact, the functions of attention and concentration are both prerequisites for any higher mental task. They set the scene for independent living, career advancement, and even social relationships.

Other complaints that go along with attention and concentration deficits are fatigue, an increased need for sleep, easy distractibility, an inability to shift from topic to topic while engaged in conversation, and a lack of focus.

Mindset #2: Initiation and Planning of Goal-Directed Activities

Interview any group of executives and you will hear them spout long-range plans, solutions to budgetary problems, and ways to implement better attitudes and health among employees. Whether or not you agree with the proposals, the fact remains that the executive can reel them off. This is a facet of what is aptly called executive function — the ability to plan, initiate, direct and monitor one's activities. But many brain-injured people have impaired executive function. Like Lorraine in the example at the beginning of this chapter, they frequently miss the point. They lack the "building block" cognitive skills needed to perform executive functions. In addition to the attention and concentration difficulties discussed earlier:

• *They may have difficulty understanding the abstract.* In other words, they're only able to take things literally. For example, George, a brain-injured teen, got into his friend Paul's car. Paul told him to put on his belt. George looked at him incredulously "I already have my belt on. Look." And he pointed to his waist where, indeed, he had a brown leather belt buckled around his pants. George didn't understand that Paul meant his seat belt.

• *Often, they can't stop talking or performing a task once they start.* A person with this particular deficit will ask the same question over and over again, making social interaction almost impossible. She might discuss a topic that had been dropped a long time before. He might continue vacuuming the living room carpet for hours until someone says, "Stop!"

• *They may have difficulty solving problems in a realistic way.* Here's an example: Mike, a brain-injured teen, decided that he wanted to go to college in the fall, but he couldn't take the necessary steps to put his plan in action. Rather than checking a college directory, sending away for bulletins, and applying to a few schools, he drove out to a nearby college on the first day of classes and asked where he should put his bags. Sally, a brain-injured adolescent in her senior year of high school, let the whole first semester slip away while she stared out her bedroom window, ready and willing to tell anyone who listened that she was going to college... soon.

• *They have difficulty keeping the steps of a task in order.* This is called a sequencing deficit. She might take a dustpan out to the garbage before sweeping the floor. He might dry the dirty pots before they are washed, if he initiates any action in the first place. Usually, brain-injured people with impairment of executive functions have difficulty initiating actions unless they're specifically asked or cued.

Mildly brain-injured people with impairment of executive functions may be unaware that anything is wrong. They blame the misplaced work, the overdue deadline, the long absences, on others. That's because they have poor deficit awareness — that is, a lack of understanding about their disability.

• *They have trouble learning from their mistakes — and their successes.* You might say this is true for all of us at one time or another, but a brain-injured person with this cognitive deficit might, say, continue to knock on his boss' door after it had been slammed in his face. Or a brain-injured teen might receive a special dessert from her mother if she had cleaned up her room, but when her mother tells her that this is a reward for a task well done, the teenager gives her a puzzled look.

Impairment of executive functions might be a common

HEADLINERS

"Looking back on this entire incident, I realize that it was the most significant and influential event of my life. As a thirteen-year-old, I had never stopped to examine everything I had. I had simply taken for granted my health, my life, and, more importantly, the lives of each member of my family. It was this incredible realization of mortality which struck me the hardest. I was surrounded by friends and relatives but I cannot remember a more intense feeling of being isolated and alone. It had taken a tragedy such as this to enable me to fully appreciate my own life...

"Of course, there were times when my parents broke down under the tremendous pressure they felt. I remember sitting in the hospital dayroom with my father, my mother, my brother, and my sister sobbing, thinking only of what Lenny meant to us. He was physically as close as the intensive care unit next door but too far away from us to make contact with him. We all shared the same feeling of helplessness, and I believe it was this that brought us so close together as a family. We became open and honest in our communication with each other. Our conversations included all the positive memories of our growing up years. We supported each other with hope and encouragement. We cried together, we laughed together, we prayed together. Most important of all, we needed each other."

"Reflections of a Brother" by Michael Burke
(Reprinted from "First Person Accounts"
from the Brain Injury Association, Inc.)

deficit, but it's not an easy one to accept. One study found that 90% of brain-injured people suffering from impairment of executive function could not handle vocational training.

Mindset #3: Judgment and Perception

This mindset gets to the very heart of thinking. Without the ability to judge or perceive a situation, people cannot analyze it. They will have trouble interpreting the actions or the intentions of others. They will be confused when he gets more than one piece of information at a time. They will "talk a good game," but there will be nothing behind their words. They will have an unrealistic appraisal of themselves, of their strengths and weaknesses. They won't be able to correct or monitor their behavior. In short, life and its struggles, its joys and its tragedies, become devoid of meaning for anything deeper than an after-dinner sweet.

Here are two examples:

Joe thinks he is the hottest thing in town, despite the fact that he's really 30 pounds overweight and in need of a shave and a job.

Alice, on the other hand, has trouble with the larger picture. When her boyfriend got sick, she kept whining that he wasn't paying enough attention to her. Soon her whining turned to anger.

These two examples also point out an outgrowth of this mindset: denial. Judgment and perception are not just necessary qualities to view the outside world — they are also necessary for self-awareness. If you can't accurately perceive or judge your situation, you'll never realize that you have a problem. One of our patients at HealthSouth RIOSA was a prominent New Jersey lawyer and amateur pilot. He had been in a car crash and suffered a brain injury Most of the damage was in the frontal areas of his brain, which lead to impairment of executive function. He could no longer practice law.

Unfortunately, he didn't believe he had any problems. He went back to his law firm and was subsequently asked to "retire." More dangerously, he tried to go up in his two-seater plane and fly solo.

Self-awareness is the ultimate function — for everyone. Teaching a brain-injured person that he is indeed disabled, and that he now has judgment and perception impairments, is a prerequisite for successful rehabilitation.

HEADLINERS

ATTENTION PLEASE!

There are two types of attention:

• Sustained attention gives you the ability to concentrate on one specific task, conversation, movie, or TV show for a specific amount of time.

• Selective attention allows you to focus on one thing while lots of other things are going on around you. A student can listen to a teacher's lecture while "tuning out" the sound of the lawn mower outside the window. A beer-bellied husband can watch the football game on TV while "tuning out" his brother-in-law's small talk. An executive can listen to a sales pitch over lunch while "tuning out" the sounds of the other diners.

We'll discuss some of the ways we teach self-awareness at HealthSouth RIOSA later on in the book.

Mindset #4: Learning and Memory

Memory problems are thought to be the result of temporal lobe damage (where most memory is stored) or damage to the hippocampus (which is responsible for registering and retrieving information). In one study, 86% of severely memory-impaired brain injury patients had hippocampal damage.

Naturally a lack of memory will hinder rehabilitation and re-entry into the community. In a different study, 65% of brain-injured persons who could not find work had memory impairment.

Memory also reflects the other mindsets. It's simple: If you cannot perceive something, you can't learn it. If you can't learn it, you can't remember it.

Here are some examples of very real problems that memory deficits create:

1. You can't remember the name of streets when you give directions to your house of many years.
2. You can never seem to find your keys or your glasses or your checkbook.
3. You can't remember people's names after you've met them several times.
4. You don't remember meeting someone you first met only a few days ago.
5. You get passed over for promotion when you return to the job because you can't seem to remember your work responsibilities.

Unfortunately, memory problems are very stubborn. Even when patients in a rehabilitation hospital were asked to repeat the hour of their therapy appointment (which was at the same time every day), it took between four and eight weeks for them to memorize this one simple fact.

Because memory is so intricately involved in day-to-day living, memory problems are among the most important to overcome. *(In Chapter Ten, we'll discuss some of the rehabilitation techniques that are used to "jog" a brain-injured person's memory.)*

Mindset #5: Speed of Information Processing

When the brainstem is injured, it can create a "slow-motion" effect. Simple tasks can take forever. A patient might remember what his name is and can even write it down — if you give him 10 minutes. She'll say goodbye to you — after you've already hung up the phone.

HEADLINERS

SEEING IS BELIEVING?

Even if a brain-injured person's five senses are intact, his problems with perception will also create sensory impairments. His hearing might be fine, but if he can't perceive that the car honking outside is waiting for him to put on his coat and leave, it doesn't much matter that he can hear every honk. He might have 20/20 vision, but if he can't perceive that the hornet he sees flying near him is going to sting him, seeing, quite literally, isn't believing.

Unfortunately, speed is of the essence in our society. Families are quick to lose their patience when dealing with this deficit. It can be extremely frustrating to wait many seconds for a loved one to respond to the simple question, "What did you do today?" When there's no immediate response, the family member may repeat the question. Still no response. While the brain-injured survivor is taking time to process the question, and struggling to remember the day's events, the other person may get irritated, thinking to herself, "He just isn't listening to me." She may compound the problem by asking a different question before he had time to respond to the first.

Mindset #6: Communication

All of us have times when it is just too hard to communicate what we want to get across. This can be an ongoing problem for the brain-injured. Their language and communication problems usually stem from damage to the left hemisphere of the brain.

Here are some examples:

She might have trouble naming an object. She knows that the door has just opened, but she cannot seem to say the word "door."

He might have difficulty remembering the word he wants to use; it will always be "on the tip of my tongue."

She might slur her words.

He might speak too slowly.

She might have had an incredible vocabulary before her car accident, one befitting the English teacher she was. But that was before. She now has a vocabulary of 20 words.

He might talk without thinking first. Lacking an inhibiting

"social censor," he'll tell the woman sitting next to him on the bus that she's "as fat as a pig." He'll tell his boss that he doesn't feel like typing any letters right now — or ever again, for that matter.

She might talk too much, without letting another person get a word in edgewise. (These last two examples involve behavioral abnormalities that affect communication.)

Communication is not just the power of speech. It's also the ability to comprehend language and to express one's thoughts and ideas — all of which can be hindered in a brain injury. The result is a "wandering mind." For example, Julie started discussing her new ad campaign with her client — only to begin talking, without skipping a beat, about the traffic en route to the city that morning. Unfortunately, the client didn't know that Julie had suffered a brain injury. He just found her odd, rude, and irritating. And he hated the campaign.

Language disorders can involve both spoken and written words. In the same way that a novice student of French may understand much of the spoken language without being able to speak it well himself, so a brain-injured person might be able to follow what you say to him but be unable to respond appropriately. Also, he might comprehend what he reads but not be capable of writing his thoughts down on paper.

These, then, are the mindsets that interfere with a person's ability to function on the job, at home, and in society at large. And, as if it weren't enough that a person can't remember a recent fact, that she can't write her name, that he can no longer think logically, cognitive problems also create *behavioral problems*. That's what we'll be looking at next.

Frustration. Irritation. Depression. Disinhibition. All these can have cognitive roots; all may be the result of brain damage. All have far-reaching consequences for a brain-injured person and for those who love him or her. Read on...

CHAPTER EIGHT

BEHAVIORAL SYMPTOMS OF BRAIN INJURY

*"I can't help it, but sometimes
I gotta wonder, 'Why me?...'"*

A 28-year-old former plant manager,
a patient at HealthSouth

• Sally was a real clotheshorse before her brain injury. She had so many outfits, shoes, and accessories that she had to have a consultant come in and help her design an organized, space-saving closet. But now she changes her clothes every single time she walks into her room, throwing the slinky black dress she wore for breakfast onto the ever-growing pile on the floor, and rifling through her closet for a ski jacket to wear for lunch.

• Milton never had a weight problem before his brain injury. He loved a good steak and fries as much as the next guy, but he worked it off in his company's gym. And, unless he was out celebrating, he only ate when he was hungry. But now he's like a speeding train, shoveling down food before it has a chance to cool on his plate. Day and night, you'll find Milton at the kitchen table or a TV table, eating anything and everything in sight.

• Since Savannah returned home from the rehabilitation hospital, she's been improving by leaps and bounds. She's never late for her therapy appointments. She eats her meals at specific times. She works hard at keeping up her personal grooming habits. But there is one problem

Savannah's mother didn't discover until the damage was done. It seemed Savannah loved the catalogs that came in the mail. She'd think nothing of picking up the phone and ordering whatever she wanted. T-shirts, a vacuum cleaner, a china pet bowl, silk flowers — you name it and Savannah charged it by phone. When the items came to the house, Savannah didn't want them anymore. Nor did she have the money to pay for them.

• George was a model husband and father before his brain injury. Conservative and upright to the core, he was considered the quintessential family man. But lately upper management has been getting some disturbing reports. George pinched several of the secretaries as they walked down the corridor. He made lewd remarks at the last sales presentation. He made a pass at a colleague. He was sexually out of control.

• Timothy was always the class clown. Ever since fifth grade, he had been a mobile comedy act. Even the teachers couldn't help but laugh at some of his antics. But after he fell off his bicycle, Timothy changed; his jokes became nasty. He told one teacher she was disgusting and fat. He told a friend that he was the biggest nerd walking on two feet. He snipped off a girl's long ponytail. And to make matters worse, he didn't shut up. All day long he talked. During class. During assemblies. During the walk to school. Soon Timothy was talking only to himself. None of his old friends would go near him. And his teachers were losing their patience.

Different ages. Different lives. Different people with

one common link: All of them were victims of brain injury. And all of them are suffering because of inappropriate behavior they can't control or understand.

AN ACT IS AN ACT IS AN ACT

Human beings function at higher levels than their animal counterparts. The fact is that we can think. We can plan long-term goals. But there's even something beyond "cognitive awareness." We humans can also *feel*.

Feelings at their most rudimentary level are common to all the higher species. Take one brainstem, some basic sensory perception equipment and decent motor function, and any animal, from a snake to a squirrel, will feel pain or contentment.

But these are feelings without perspective. Only humans can *interpret* their feelings. And only humans have the cognitive ability to control their emotions. A woman who has just broken up with her fiancé is in tears, but she must muster her self-control because she has an important business meeting in half an hour. A man is furious when a taxi driver slams into his car. He gets out, ready to fight, until he sees that the taxi driver is over six feet tall and built like Arnold Schwarzenegger.

These are only two small examples, but they show that cognitive abilities and emotions are closely aligned. Just as cognitive functions are vulnerable to brain injury, so are the emotions and the ways they make people behave. In fact, there are three facets to the behavioral symptoms of brain injury, three "hats" that can play havoc with emotions, behavior and life in the world at large:

HAT #1: Neurological Damage

In Chapter One, you learned how most neurotransmitters in the brain inhibit behavior. When the delicate balance of neurotransmitters is disrupted, they can no longer do their job. Your emotional balance gets upset; you may suddenly say things that formerly you might have only thought, or you might act with the emotional immaturity of a young child.

Unfortunately most of the inhibiting neurotransmitters inhabit the frontal and temporal lobes, which, as you now know, are often damaged in a brain injury.

One reason behavioral problems rear their head is that brain-injured survivors no longer have the cognitive skills to perceive, understand, plan, or communicate appropriately. Without an apparatus for logic, Sally, the clotheshorse, won't know that she shouldn't wear an evening gown to breakfast. Without a perceptive social censor, George doesn't realize that his sexual advances are inappropriate. Without the ability to recognize that he is full (or the memory that he has just eaten), Milton can consume food at an astounding rate. Here's another brain injury fact:

Damaged or deficient neurotransmitters combined with a lack of cognitive skills translates into inappropriate behavior.

But neurological damage is only one-third of the story.

HAT #2: Reactionary Disturbances

When a brain-injured person first awakens from a coma, he may be agitated and confused. Think about it. Here he is in a strange hospital room, lying in a strange bed without a clue as to how he got there, or, in some cases, who he is.

Later, as he becomes more oriented, his agitation will turn to general irritability, which can last for days, months, or, in some cases, until the day he dies. This irritability comes from frustration; he can't do the simple tasks he'd always done before. Writing a check becomes a long, involved chore. Going to the supermarket is so complicated that it is impossible. Driving the kids to school can never be done again; he can't remember where the school is.

Sometimes irritability goes hand in hand with denial. As we have seen in Chapter Seven, denial can have a neurological base (*anosognosia*). But denial can also have a life of its own, as a psychological reaction to the injury. A patient might become defensive whenever his limitations are pointed out. He might get belligerent when he discovers that his old goals are impossible to achieve. He might refuse to acknowledge his impairments, becoming angry and withdrawn when he can't do something. In full-blown denial, a patient will protect his old sense of self at any cost, making rehabilitation almost impossible.

In time, most patients do come to terms with their new limitations. Unfortunately, this new awareness can trigger yet another type of reaction. Without proper rehabilitation and good outside support, it sometimes becomes the springboard for drug and alcohol abuse, withdrawal, or even suicide.

Of course, we're talking about *depression*. Though it's sometimes the product of a chemical imbalance, depression can also be a reaction to a new and frightening reality. A patient might feel incompetent and worthless, hopeless and helpless. Occasionally these negative feelings so overwhelm a brain-injured patient that nothing can help; nothing can break through the pain. Dr. Kurt Goldstein called this aura of complete and utter despair a *catastrophic reaction*.

Fortunately, most brain-injured survivors have a milder

HEADLINERS

Myth: Problem behavior in the brain-injured patient always gets better with time.

Unfortunately, it may be the other way around. A study of relatives of brain-injured patients revealed that during the first six months after the injury, the relatives noted a minimal amount of psychological problems such as depression, irritability, or anger. During the second six months, however, there was an increase in these psychological problems. It was within this time period that most patients tried to adjust to normal life. They tried to re-enter the community or the work force, and found that they were not welcome. They also became aware of their new limitations. During the third six-month period, many of these same patients had withdrawn socially; they chose isolation rather than try to overcome the negative aspects of their environment.

Another study interviewed the families of brain-injured patients at yearly intervals. The results? At one year they felt their loved one had undergone significant personality changes. They were more excitable, more irritable — or completely unemotional. At two years, their loved ones were still irritable, but now they were also inclined to act out in socially inappropriate ways. After five years, these families were still citing behavioral problems as the worst result of their loved one's accident.

form of depression, but it is painful nonetheless. Some of the signs are:

• *Psychosomatic pain.* He complains about the ache in his leg, the pounding in his brain, but there is no evidence of anything physically wrong.

• *A general loss of self-esteem.* When she realizes that she cannot organize her thoughts the way she once did, she feels less of a person. She hates the way she looks, the way she talks, even the way she now holds a knife and fork.

• *Mood swings.* One moment he'll be crying at a welcome-home party; the next, he'll be screaming at his wife for cooking a dish he hates.

• *Anxiety.* She is filled with nervous tension. She can't help it. Ever since she became aware of her limitations, she has been afraid — of people laughing at the way she speaks, of dressing wrong, of being unemployed, of not being able to handle a purchase at the five-and-dime, of being alone, unloved, and unwanted.

• *Sleep disturbances.* A study by Dr. George Prigatano et. al. discovered that brain-injured survivors woke up more during the night and had fewer deep sleep cycles than their healthy counterparts. This lack of balanced, rhythmic sleep can create more depression — as well as irritability and anxiety.

• *Suicidal thoughts.* A study of depressed brain-injured World War II soldiers found that the risk of suicide was still present 15 to 20 years after the injury. The possibility always exists. Listen to your brain-injured loved one. Watch him. At the first sign of danger, contact your physician.

Brain injury is a devastating trauma. The way a person reacts to it will be no less dramatic. The loss of your friends, of your place in the family sphere, of your career, your wishes and aspirations, of that person you once were and knew so well — all these cause strong emotional reactions: anger, depression, irritability, and more. And because there are usually cognitive deficits at work as well, these reactions will usually appear in disruptive, socially inappropriate — and sometimes dangerous — ways.

HAT #3: Pre-Existing Conditions

In a strange way, brain-injured survivors sometimes become more of what they were. For example, someone who abused alcohol or drugs before his brain injury will probably try to cope with his new limitations in the same way. One particular study of brain-injured patients who had a prior history of substance abuse or sexual promiscuity discovered that in most cases the injury, far from improving the situation, actually amplified pre-existing problems.

For example, Margo, a pretty 20-year-old single woman, suffered a brain injury in a car accident. After months of rehabilitation, she was sent back home to live with her frail, elderly parents. Almost at once, Margo began to act in socially inappropriate ways. She began to dress more provocatively than she had in the past, with plunging necklines, too tight clothes, and underwear as outerwear. She began to spend much of her time out of the house. Her parents were worried sick; they had no idea how to handle her. But when Margo's social worker questioned them, they admitted that Margo had become sexually active at a very early age; she had always dated several men at the same time. She was acting the way she always had, but more dramatically.

Whether they're the result of neurological damage, a reaction to an unfriendly world, or a magnification of pre-existing conditions, behavioral symptoms are hard to take — for everyone. But forewarned is forearmed. You now know something of the general symptoms of depression, agitation, and irritability. In order to better recognize other, more specific signs of inappropriate behavior, read on.

1. "Get Out of My Room!" or Verbal Outbursts

Verbal outbursts are unpleasant, especially if you're on the receiving end. They explode, as if out of nowhere, but the patient soon forgets them. Verbal outbursts stem from a faulty limbic system — the area of the brain responsible for emotional states — and can occur sporadically throughout the brain-injured survivor's life.

Oddly enough, these verbal outbursts rarely take place after major crises. Rather, the patient will lash out at the minor, insignificant stresses of daily life: a misplaced key, a person in the "8 items or less" checkout lane with 12 items in the cart, a neighborhood dog walking on their lawn.

Believe it or not, there's an explanation for these outbursts. Small, insignificant situations are the very ones the patient would have handled without a thought in the past. But now, every one of these actions, every one of these situations may uncover his inability to deal with simple stress and frustration.

Another point: How you react to these outbursts will greatly influence the brain-injured person's behavior. Do your best to stay calm and speak in a soothing voice; redirect the person quickly by changing the topic and finding a quiet, distraction-free environment. It's important to reward appropriate behavior, but not punish for verbal outbursts. For example, a decrease in verbal punishment might be rewarded with increased television or a movie, while continued outbursts are met with no reward. Reinforce the positive!

2. "Breaking Down the House" or Physical Outbursts

Throwing an ashtray, breaking a vase, or hurling spaghetti against the wall can be triggered by events that normally would not cause such behavior. Brain-injured survivors have difficulty controlling their impulses. Noisy, chaotic and frustrating circumstances tend to increase the chance that such an outburst may occur. These outbursts are not premeditated but are more like an "automatic reflex."

3. "I'm Most Important" or Egocentricity

Your brain-injured loved one has indeed gone through a terrible experience, and he needs to talk about himself, about the pain he's been through, to release some of that tension. But his egocentricity can also be a product of paranoia, of an inability to make a connection between logic and reality. Think of it. What if you lacked the ability to understand what someone was saying? What if you couldn't use your logic to realize that someone *really* isn't talking about you, or isn't trying to "get you?" All your focus would be on yourself. You would demand the attention of others. You would be completely unaware of other people's problems. And you would be functionally unable to share anything with anyone.

But egocentricity can hurt. One study found that a

brain-injured survivor's social network usually disintegrates after about six months, just enough time for friends to have new experiences that don't involve their brain-injured pal, just enough time for them to see that their friend has become an angry, depressed individual who only wants to talk about himself and who doesn't care about them at all.

4. "Everything You've Always Wanted to Know About..." or Sexual Problems

Freud always claimed it was always on people's minds. But whether or not the idea of sex is a constant companion in everyday life, the libido is most definitely a factor in brain injury. Sex drive may either increase or decrease. Some men's testosterone levels drop. Some women stop menstruating. These symptoms can have their roots in neurological damage to the hypothalamus (the regulator of sexual drive) or in purely psychological reactions. But cause isn't as important as result. The fact is that 50% or more of brain-injured adults experience some form of sexual disturbance that sabotages their attempts to re-enter the real world.

Most brain injuries occur to people under 25 — in other words, to adolescents who are still developing, physically, mentally, and sexually. They are in a state of confusion; their hormones are surging. Add to this energetic libido the fact that many of these same brain-injured teens come from unstable, unsupportive homes, and you have all the necessary ingredients for sexual dysfunction.

Many medications are given to brain-injured survivors to prevent seizures, control blood pressure, or improve behavior. But they may also decrease feelings of sexuality or even cause impotence.

Role reversal also dampens sexuality between partners. What if your husband, who was always the one to handle the family's crises, large and small, became dependent after a head injury? You, the wife, may discover that being a 24-hour caregiver takes much of the thrill out of sex. Or what if it was your wife who was injured, and this formerly independent, accomplished woman now whines louder than your kids? These family dynamics need to be addressed before frustration, anger, and bitterness displace tenderness and love. Rehabilitation hospitals can help; so can family therapists. Don't be afraid to ask for help. The problem is much more common than you might think.

Compounding sexual dysfunction are the cognitive deficits that prevent a brain-injured man or woman from

---

HEADLINERS

ONE GIRL'S STORY

Jeanette never liked herself much; her self-esteem had never been high. But as she grew up, she discovered that by doing things for others, from donating to charity to being a thoughtful friend, she could actually find herself likeable. But after her brain injury, Jeanette couldn't do the things that made her feel good about herself. Consequently, her self-esteem plummeted. She felt worthless. All the negative feelings that had been under wraps before the accident came out in full bloom. She became extremely depressed.

correctly interpreting cues, sexual or otherwise. Picture this scenario: A brain-injured man needing a bath and a shampoo goes to a singles' bar looking for a date. In his mind, he looks really terrific; he can't understand why the women are ignoring him. Instead of feeling good about his night on the town, he becomes anxious, frustrated, and depressed.

Here's another scenario: A young brain-injured woman believes the line a handsome young man gives her. She's in love, he tells her he loves her, too. But he dumps her after a one-night stand, and she can't understand why. She begins to hate herself; she gets depressed and withdrawn. It had to be something she did wrong.

On a different note, here's a story that connects sexuality with memory. One patient insisted on having sex with his wife 8, 10, 12 times a day When he came back home from the hospital, she couldn't get any of her chores done. It wasn't the fact that the man was insatiable. In reality, he had such severe short-term memory as a result of his brain injury that he didn't remember having sex!

5. "I'm Right and There's No Use Arguing" or Rigidity and Inflexibility

As with most behavioral problems, rigidity and inflexibility have cognitive roots. Difficulty with problem solving, reasoning and behavior often result in rigid and inflexible thinking and behavior. A brain-injured person might be incapable of switching from one topic of conversation to another. His memory could be so poor that he is completely unaware that he's mentioned the same subject four times in the last five minutes. He might obsessively talk about a particular idea or concept for weeks at a time. Without the ability to think of multiple solutions to a single problem, the patient is "stuck" with a single, inflexible course to follow.

6. *"Look Before You Leap" or Impulsive Behavior*

"Think before you act" has no meaning to a brain-injured person with an impulse-control problem. When the inhibiting neurotransmitters get damaged, a person's "social censor" — the ability to control oneself — flies out the window. Impulsivity mushrooms with stress, especially when the patient has to make a decision about something. She might "fly off the handle" at her husband when he asks her if she wants dinner now... She might type an entire five-page report only to discover that she's misspelled a word on page two. Rather than salvage what she's done, she rips up the whole report and starts from scratch... She might decide to go up to the apartment of a man she just met on the bus, even though she knows nothing about him. It just seems like a good idea.

But there's still one aspect to behavior we have yet to explore. It's the single most important trait a brain-injured person can have, but it's also one of the hardest to achieve...

7. *"Who Am I?" or Developing Self-Awareness*

Family Member: He just isn't the same person he was before.

Injured Person: I don't know what she's talking about. I'm still me.

Family Member: He acts so crazy at times.

Injured Person: I'm not crazy — she is.

Two different points of view, and each person feels he is right. But, unfortunately, there is no right or wrong. It all comes down to perception. The family member is frustrated that the person she once loved has not only changed, he isn't even aware of it. Her brain-injured spouse, however, is acting quite normal for someone in his condition. For him, self-awareness doesn't come easy — or fast. Not only is denial at work, but cognitive deficits as well. Listen to this sobering report:

A study of brain-injured patients and their families seven years after the initial trauma found that the families felt their brain-injured member was immature, childish, and unwilling to admit to any deficits.

But self-awareness is possible, as this woman's personal account from a Brain Injury Association, Inc. article shows:

"For me, as for most people who have sustained a head injury, knowing what was made it difficult to accept what is. I had to learn to find a way to change that which should not be accepted, but also to compromise and accept that which could not be changed."

This woman learned self-awareness, and she is only one of thousands who have also succeeded in their quest. But they couldn't learn self-awareness on their own. They needed the help of a good rehabilitation program.

HARD, AIN'T IT HARD

Rehabilitation is probably the hardest thing that your loved one will ever do. It's harder work than preparing a paper for a conference. It's harder work than taking care of three kids. It's harder work than lifting weights and toting barges. It involves physical, emotional, and mental therapy. But, as the expression goes, you don't get something for nothing. Rehabilitation can be extremely rewarding for everyone — you, your loved one, and even society at large.

The good news is that rehabilitation programs today take behavioral and emotional problems into account. *(We'll discuss some of the newest techniques in Chapter Eleven.)*

You now know how brain injuries are caused. You know what happens when a brain injury occurs. And you understand the symptoms that go beyond a "simple" bump on the head.

It's time now to talk about recovery, to find the reality behind your hope. It's time to journey toward getting well.

CHAPTER NINE

HOW TO PICK THE RIGHT REHABILITATION HOSPITAL

*"Defeat is worse than death because
you have to live with defeat."*
Bill Musselman, from 1,911 Best
Things Anybody Ever Said

MYTH: *One rehabilitation hospital is as good as the next.*

MYTH: *If you don't have any funds, forget about rehabilitation for a loved one.*

MYTH: *My husband wants to go to a rehabilitation hospital, but I think he's just trying to get attention, like he always does.*

MYTH: *My husband and I can take care of our brain-injured child just fine at home by ourselves, thank you.*

MYTH: *My wife is severely brain injured. There's no hope for her. We might as well just give up.*

If someone you love has had a brain injury, chances are you've heard some of these comments or you might even have said them yourself. It's understandable. With approximately 500 rehabilitation programs in the United States alone, there's a dizzying array of rehabilitation hospitals to choose from. Yet the family stress level may be so high that making the right decision seems an impossibility.

The fact is that good rehabilitation hospitals have been proven to really help. In a world where 80% of people with brain injuries recover their physical functions within a year but have lingering cognitive, behavioral, emotional, and social problems, good rehabilitation programs are needed more than ever. Above all, you need to know how to choose a rehabilitation hospital that meets your specifications.

THE 15 STEPS

All of us hope to function at our fullest potential, and brain-injured survivors are no exception to that rule. They deserve a comprehensive rehabilitation program. The elements of that program may be as individual as the person himself, but we believe there are 15 components that, ideally, a brain-injury rehabilitation program should include:

1. Evaluation and assessment of a patient's needs.

2. Physical independence activities dealing with mobility, strength, and endurance.

3. Activities of daily living such as dressing, grooming, personal hygiene, and feeding.

4. Cognitive rehabilitation to compensate for deficits in attention, memory, judgment, initiation, and planning.

5. Treatment for swallowing disorders.

6. Speech and language therapy for communication disorders.

7. Behavioral management and modification.

8. Sexuality counseling and support.

9. Social skills groups.

10. Family counseling to deal with adjustment to a loved one's disability.

11. Therapeutic recreation for teaching leisure skills.

12. Vocational assessment and retraining.

13. Re-entry into the community.

14. Patient and family education.

15. Alumni and support groups.

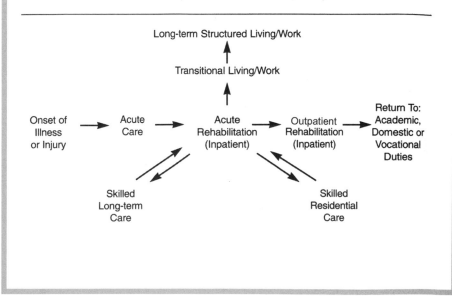

THE RECOVERY TREE

This diagram shows the possibilities
for care and rehabilitation of a brain-injured person.

To further separate the myths from the realities of rehabilitation, here are a few more things to look for in a good program:

HOME, UNCOMFORTABLE HOME

The best intentions don't always yield the best results. As much as you'd like to take care of your loved one in the privacy of your home, it's a lot tougher than you think. Would you know how to get your husband into the shower? Could you change his clothes when he soiled them? How would you handle his excessive talking or a violent outburst?

Like it or not, you should know that home is not always the best place to be after a brain-injury. First of all, a hospital setting can supply the medical attention your loved one may need. An acute-care unit will stop infection from spreading and reduce the brain swelling and pressure buildup that can cause even more damage than the original injury.

Secondly, a rehabilitation hospital employs a staff that is specifically trained in brain-injury rehabilitation. They can supply the testing, the diagnoses, and the treatment program that you just don't have at home. They will also provide the facilities and structure — from physical therapy equipment to group social skills therapy — that your loved one needs for support, retraining, and, most importantly, successful re-entry into the community.

Above all, a good rehabilitation hospital will help train you so that when your loved one is returned home, you will be better able to cope with any aberrant behavior, functional problems, and stress that you may be feeling yourself.

TYPES OF CARE

Acute Care

This is given in a regular hospital where a person usually goes immediately following a brain injury. It will most likely have an emergency room, operating room, and intensive care unit.

Acute Inpatient Rehabilitation

This is usually a freestanding rehabilitation hospital, although it may be a unit in an acute-care hospital. It should provide a complete interdisciplinary team and designated brain-injury program, supplying all of the components described in this book.

Outpatient Rehabilitation (Day Treatment)

The survivor will live at home but come to the rehab center daily for a four- to eight-hour structured therapy program. It should have clearly defined components for vocational and community re-entry in addition to the usual therapies.

Transitional Living Center

This may be a house, group of apartments, campus setting, or ranch. The survivor lives in a structured environment where the necessary therapies can be provided. The goal is greater independence, but supervision, safety, and support are very much at hand. The brain-injured survivor might attend school or have a job.

Skilled Long-Term Care

Lower-level patients who cannot be cared for at home may require placement in a skilled nursing facility, a group home, or nursing home. Many facilities have therapists on staff or who visit the facility daily.

Knowing how to take care of a brain-injured survivor will also help continue his rehabilitation — which doesn't stop when he does come home.

REFERENCES UPON REQUEST

Never underestimate the value of a recommendation. If your family doctor, a man or woman you trust, suggests a rehabilitation hospital, check it out. Other ways to get recommendations are:

1. By contacting HealthSouth at One HealthSouth Parkway, Birmingham, Alabama 35243 (800) 765-4772 or at www.healthsouth.com.
2. Through your health or disability insurance company.
3. Through your firm's human resources department.
4. Through social workers in your area.
5. Through other families within your community who have gone through the same experience as you.
6. By contacting the Brain Injury Association at 105 North Alfred Street, Alexandria, VA 22314, 703 236-6000 or (800) 444-6443.

YOU DESERVE THE BEST

Not all programs are the same. In the same way you'd seek a second opinion if you needed an operation, so should you research rehabilitation hospitals. Although location is a factor, it shouldn't be the deciding one. It may be well worth the effort to travel that extra 100 miles or so for a program that offers exceptional service.

Try to get the names of some other families who have

gone through the program at a particular hospital. Call or write them. See if their needs were similar to yours. Ask them what they were looking for in a program when their loved one was injured and if they are pleased with the rehabilitation hospital they chose. Another telling point: Ask them if they would do anything differently if they could start over again.

ONE VISIT IS WORTH A THOUSAND WORDS

Let's face it: A rehabilitation hospital's brochure is going to put its best foot forward. How many of us have seen a hotel's lush brochure, complete with palm trees, ocean-view balconies, and spacious rooms, only to arrive and discover the cramped, slightly seedy reality?

But seeing is believing and we cannot stress this enough:

VISIT ANY PROSPECTIVE FACILITY

Use your eyes. Inspect the rooms, the offices, the therapy areas. Make sure that the hospital is clean, and that there is sufficient space for all the different types of therapy that must be done to meet rehabilitation goals. Watch the staff. Are they attentive to their patients? Do they know where each patient should be at all times? Do the patients themselves have a schedule that they can follow, that, despite their deficits, has been taught to them in some form?

DOCTOR, DOCTOR

The caring doctors on "ER" may be figments of the scriptwriter's imagination, but as busy and inundated with paperwork as today's doctors are, they do not have to be the Invisible Man or Woman. Meet the doctor in charge of the

HEADLINERS

Why do you walk
The way that you do?
And why do you talk
But words are so few?
I don't understand your behaviors

Why can't you call
And just dial the phone?
In fact, I'm appalled
You can't live alone.
I don't understand your behaviors

Why do you toil
When baking a cake?
Can't measure the foil?
You're so hard to take!
I don't understand your behaviors

Just stop acting crazy
Straighten up now
Perhaps you've turned lazy?
But sweat's on your brow
I don't understand your behaviors
Angry at me?
What did I do?
Oh, I failed to see
Beyond bodily clues
Teach me... to perceive
your behaviors

A Poem by Janice Cortis Kasowski,
as reprinted in "First Person Accounts"
from The Brain Injury Association, Inc.

facilities. If you were investigating HealthSouth RIOSA, you would make an appointment to meet with me, Richard Senelick. As Medical Director, I make it a policy to meet all interested families, and I answer any of their questions to the best of my ability. I know that if I were in their shoes, I'd want the same respect.

Not just the doctor, but also the staff may be interviewed and questioned. Don't be afraid to ask them about their credentials and experience. How accessible are they? Do they seem sensitive to your needs? Do they treat their patients with compassion? Does the hospital use a team approach, in which cognitive retraining, behavioral therapies, social skills training, vocational and physical therapies are all equally stressed with everyone working together?

MONEY WON'T BUY EVERYTHING, IT'S TRUE

Finances are always the bottom line. But bottom lines can be explored, analyzed, and understood. The rehabilitation hospitals you are checking out should have case managers who will be individually handling your insurance matters. They will keep you informed about progress, financial resources, insurance payments, and the exact cost of the program over and above what is paid by insurance. In their article "Advocating for Funds," The Brain Injury Association suggests that financial assistance may also be obtained from such public programs as Supplemental Security Income (SSI), the Social Services Block Grant, Veteran's Benefits, and Vocational Rehabilitation. Private sources include Workers' Compensation, Auto No-Fault and Liability, Accident and Health Insurance, Preferred Provider Organizations, Health Maintenance Organizations, Short- and Long-Term Disability, Reinsurance and Self-Insurance, as well as funds from private philanthropic organizations.

DRUG DEALING

It's sad, but true. As we have seen throughout this book, drug and alcohol abuse go hand in hand with brain injury. Make sure that your rehabilitation hospital of choice has access to support groups to help patients deal with substance abuse, and that it offers patients more positive ways to cope, including relaxation strategies and the solid support of peers. Further, the rehabilitation program should also incorporate a behavior and environment management program in which drugs are locked up to keep the patients' surroundings safe.

A FAMILY AFFAIR

Illness is never a solitary pursuit. Whether it's a broken leg, major depression, or a brain injury, the patient's family (or close-knit circle of friends) will always be involved. Make sure that the rehabilitation hospital includes you in the treatment team, explaining procedures, medical terminology, and prognosis for recovery. Find out if family therapy or meetings are routinely scheduled, and if the staff teaches you as well as the patient. After all, you will ultimately be the responsible caregiver.

INSTINCTIVE BEHAVIOR

When it comes to childrearing, the famed Dr. Spock had said, "Trust your instincts." The same goes for your brain-injured loved one and the rehabilitation facility you ultimately choose. Trust your feelings. Observe how welcome the place makes you feel, how professional the staff appears, how clean, safe, and efficient the surroundings are, how the staff

HEADLINERS

REHABILITATION CHECKLIST

Some questions to help you in your rehabilitation search:

❑ *Will the family receive regular reports on the patient's progress?*

❑ *How many people with brain injury has the center treated?*

❑ *What is the average length of stay? Who determines it?*

❑ *Are previous medical records incorporated into evaluations and treatment?*

❑ *Can the family participate in therapies?*

❑ *If the family lives far away, how much telephone contact is there?*

❑ *How often are comprehensive re-evaluations performed?*

❑ *How does the center feel about medication?*

❑ *Can the center meet the injured person's specific and individual needs, including feeding tube, bowel and bladder control, loss of vision, language therapies, group therapies, and more?*

❑ *Is there follow-up after discharge? How often?*

treats you, your loved one, and other patients. It's true that you will need education in caring for a brain-injured loved one, but don't underestimate the power of love. It can go far.

But there's more. In order to fully understand a rehabilitation facility, you need to know exactly who is on staff and why. We'll review this next.

CHAPTER TEN

THE TREATMENT TEAM

*"I don't think of her as my physical therapist.
I think of her as my friend."*
*A 36-year-old housewife and patient
at HealthSouth RIOSA*

• The physical therapist lifts his arm slowly and helps him maneuver from the wheelchair to the rocker for vestibular stimulation.

• The occupational therapist helps her become more aware, providing education and training in tasks of daily living including oral hygiene, grooming, and dressing.

• The speech therapist puts her hands on either side of her mouth, helping to promote oral muscle activity.

These are descriptions of rehabilitation in action. Physical therapists, occupational therapists, speech therapists and others all work together to provide the best possible care and treatment for brain-injured patients.

But, as you could tell when you read over these statements, rehabilitation can sound rather complex and uninviting. You already know how to pick a good facility. Now it's time to actually enter the maze and discover the cast of characters who work in concert to help your loved one as best they can.

THE MEMBERS OF THE TEAM

The Captain: The Rehabilitation Physician

A neurologist specializes in disorders of the nervous

system, specifically the spinal cord and the brain. A physiatrist is a doctor of physical medicine and rehabilitation. In addition to treating medical problems, these doctors might also oversee the rehabilitation hospital's physical, occupational, and speech therapists. Either or both doctors may direct the medical and rehabilitation care of the brain-injured patient including the management of medications.

Pitcher: The Neuropsychologist

Neuropsychologists specialize in the relationship between the brain and behavior. They perform those numerous neuropsychological tests we discussed in Chapter Five, as well as evaluate a patient's cognitive abilities, his behavior, and any psychological problems he might have. This information will be passed along to the entire team — as well as to the patient and his family — to help determine a specific rehabilitation program.

They also conduct group and support therapies, as well as individual and family therapy. These therapies frequently involve the establishment of a behavior management program.

First Basemen: Physical Therapists

Their function is exactly as it sounds: to treat the brain-injured person's physical deficits. This might mean teaching the patient to:

- Walk again
- Use a wheelchair on various terrains
- Get in and out of a wheelchair
- Maintain normal posture

Physical therapists also work on improving muscle tone, flexibility, balance, coordination, movement, energy endurance, and strength through various exercises and activities. They will work closely with the other "basemen."

Second Basemen: Occupational Therapists

The picture most people see when they envision occupational therapists at work is supervising a room full of hospital-robed patients making pottery vases and potholders. In reality, occupational therapists are involved in every aspect of a brain-injured patient's rehabilitation. Finger and hand agility. Perception. Cognitive functioning. Eye-hand coordination. Activities of daily living (ADL) functioning, relearning everything from how to take a bath to how to cut a steak. All these and more are the province of occupational therapists. And, oh yes, in improving social interaction and thought processes within groups, occupational therapists just might have some pottery sessions.

Shortstops: Speech Therapists

Speech therapists know a lot more than how to correct a lisp. Responsibilities include evaluating and treating deficits in the areas of speech production, language expression, comprehension, reading, writing, and even swallowing. They are also key players in the rehabilitation of cognitive functioning, working on the patient's attention and memory skills as well as his skills in abstract reasoning and decision making. In addition, speech therapists pay attention to social skills, helping the brain-injured patient re-master the art of conversation. Finally, since behavior and cognition are so interrelated, speech therapists often assist in developing and implementing the patient's behavior management program.

Third Basemen: Rehabilitation Nurses

Nurses are key players in any hospital program, and rehabilitation nurses have a particularly vital function. They tend to the patient's needs and comforts, but that's the beginning. In addition, they help evaluate and treat his physical health, his problems with personal hygiene, and his impaired bladder and bowel control. They pass along their information to the attending physicians and the other members of the team. They're involved in helping the patient reach his therapy goals during non-therapy hours. (For example, if the physical therapist is teaching the patient how to transfer himself into and out of his wheelchair, the nurse will help him practice his transfers in the evenings.) Nurses also play an important role in social skills training, such as helping the patient relearn to eat, mingle socially, and function with others.

Outfielders: Respiratory Therapists

Unless a patient is severely brain-injured, these therapists may only be involved in the early stages of recovery. They will be on call if the patient has trouble breathing or coughing, or needs tracheotomy care. The expert care of respiratory therapists frequently prevents infection and complications.

Outfielders: Clinical Dietitians

Everyone has to eat right — including brain-injured patients. Dietitians are especially important for them because nutritional needs can change drastically after an accident. Injured people might have lost a great deal of weight in the early stages of recovery, especially if they were in a coma; they will need more food to help their physical recuperation. Dietitians will also detail a diet for those brain-injured survivors who cannot control their eating, as well as special diets for those with bowel or swallowing problems.

Outfielders: Vocational Specialists

Independence is the goal of any good rehabilitation program. In order for brain-injured people to achieve a sense of independence and self-esteem, they must learn to live in the outside world. That's where vocational specialists come in. If the patient is a student, they will evaluate his academic performance, develop an individualized education "package" for him, and help place him in a school when the time comes.

If the patient is an adult, vocational specialists will help her with career goals. They will work with the speech therapist to build up attention and concentration skills, cooperativeness, the ability to follow directions, and more. They will teach specific job skills, from typing and hairdressing to sewing and welding, if the patient is unable to return to the job she held before the accident.

Outfielders: Rehabilitation Counselors

Like neuropsychologists, rehabilitation counselors deal with the psychological and behavioral ramifications of a brain-injured patient. But rehab counselors are also involved in the patient's social behavior and his history. These counselors interview both the patient and his family, asking detailed questions about the patient's personality before the trauma, his habits, his education, and his development. The rehab counselors' assessments analyze the family structure as well as the family's goals for their loved one. This assessment helps the staff and family work together; it helps both of them with long-term hopes and goals.

Outfielders: Recreational Activities

Leisure time is as important as work, and leisure time can also be educational. Recreational activities help patients re-enter their community. Field trips can be initiated to, say, supermarkets or restaurants. Group events can be organized, such as gardening, cooking, arts and crafts, or music appreciation. All of these activities provide opportunities for patients to practice new or relearned skills in functional, real-life situations. Recreational activities also help patients use community resources, such as public transportation or the public library, to help make re-entry into the real world as smooth as possible.

Team Organizers: Case Managers

The glue that holds the pieces together. The mechanism that turns the wheel. The umbrella that deflects the rain. Case managers are all these and more. They are the liaison between the patient and his family and the insurance company, and always on an ongoing and dynamic basis. Case managers explain to families what their loved one's rehabilitation program hopes to accomplish. They help the family find financial resources to pay for rehabilitation. They also help the family find support groups to deal with their own stress. They continue to assist the patient and his family over the long haul, helping the family cope with the patient's re-entry into the community. In short, whenever the family

---

HEADLINERS

REHABILITATION STAFFERS ARE PEOPLE, TOO

There's no doubt about it. Working with a brain-injured patient can be frustrating. Inappropriate remarks, emotional mood swings, confusion, cognitive failings — all these can take their toll. As any family member knows, you need time out, too.

The staff must make a commitment not only to help a patient, but to help themselves as well. Social support systems. Staff social functions. Staff meetings to let off "steam." Plus further education to:

- *Keep themselves stimulated*
- *Help the patients even more*
- *Remind themselves of why they wanted to enter the rehabilitation field in the first place: to help someone in need.*

---

has a problem, a question, or a concern, their first stop is the case manager. Good rehabilitation hospitals have a case manager assigned to every patient.

Player of the Year: You

Above all, there is you — the family. As the people closest to the brain-injured patient, you are the most influential and important team member of all. You should be included in all major decisions and aspects of the rehabilitation program, not just for your own sake, but also for your brain-injured loved one. Your feedback and information will help the health professionals do their job better.

A TEAM APPROACH

The baseball analogy might be stretching it, but the fact remains that every member of the team works together in an interdisciplinary approach. A baseball game isn't played by one person alone, nor can a successful rehabilitation program be carried out single-handedly.

For example, several therapists may address the patient's sequencing skills in different ways, with everyone working toward a common goal. The physical therapist helps him with the sequencing skills he needs in order to transfer himself from bed to wheelchair and wheelchair to bed. The occupational therapist helps him with the sequencing skills involved in preparing a meal. The speech therapist helps him in sequencing words and sentences to write a letter.

Another type of treatment is called co-treatment. This involves two therapists working together with a patient during a single treatment session to achieve a common goal. Co-treatment can enhance the patient's level of functioning by simultaneously addressing many deficits that interfere with her ability to perform. For example, at meal time, if the patient has trouble staying awake and also has episodes of choking, then her co-treatment might involve both a physical therapist and a speech therapist. The physical therapist would help her to sit upright with proper balance and head control, which would raise her level of alertness and make her less likely to choke. Simultaneously, the speech therapist would coach her in safe, efficient swallowing techniques.

HEADLINERS

*AN EXAMPLE OF HOW A REHABILITATION NURSE
CONTINUES THERAPY GOALS:*

Activity: Feeding

Considerations: Ensure that the patient is in an adequate **position** before **feeding** to facilitate good **swallowing**. Set up food for visual field work and one-sided neglects.

Activity: Dressing

Considerations: Ensure room is set up so patient can **find** clothing easily. Have patient **pick out clothing and organize** what they will wear that day. Start clothing on affected side and assist patient to **use the unaffected arm** to pull clothing up. Help **sequence** through activity.

Activity: Grooming

Considerations: This activity provides **tactile self-stimulation** and increases body awareness when the patient is assisted through the **task**.

Note: Interdisciplinary goals are in boldface.

THERAPY BY ANY OTHER NAME

In addition to the team approach and co-treatment, there is also intensive one-on-one therapy. Physical and occupational therapists might work alone for a concentrated dose of coordination and muscle strength; they use a lot of mat work and stretching. The speech therapist works alone in a distraction-free environment to improve attention and decrease distractibility, or to focus on specific cognitive or communication skills with the patient.

STRENGTH IN NUMBERS

Groups can sometimes accomplish what individuals alone cannot. There is strength in numbers plus peer pressure and understanding. Therefore, group therapy is another approach often used to:

- Offer valuable support among others in the same situation.
- Help develop social skills.
- Create empathy and sympathy, two strong feelings that will help the patient re-enter the community.
- Facilitate awareness of deficits by observing and critiquing others with similar problems.

From the case manager to the dietitian, this is the rehabilitation team you and your loved one will get to know well. But there's still more. Before you can freely walk through the rehabilitation maze, you must understand the process. Read on.

CHAPTER ELEVEN

THE PROCESS OF REHABILITATION

"The sooner you get someone into the rehab setting, the more you can help them regain some level of independence."
Mary Ann, R.N., at HealthSouth RIOSA

You didn't think it could happen. You never gave it another thought. Brain injuries occur to other people, other lives. But it did happen. You went camping with your family that vacation weekend. You couldn't sleep that first night. You crept out of your sleeping bag. You crawled out of the tent, carefully, silently, so you would not wake your family. You stared at the dying embers of the fire. You put on your hiking shoes and walked to the left, to the appealing stretch of trees and starlit night. You were looking for the Big Dipper when your foot slipped. You reached the end of the path; the edge of the cliff awaited. You felt stunned and surprised, barely uttering a word, until you hit the bottom. Your head struck a rock...

Next you hear the sirens above the cliff. You see a whirring red light. But where are you? What are those lights? Who are you?

You lose consciousness again. You are taken to the emergency ward of a nearby hospital. Your spouse sits next to your bed, holding your hand and crying. Your children are outside. But you are still unconscious, unaware or not sure of where you are, who you are, and what happened to bring you to this place.

What happens to millions of people every year has also

happened to you. You have had a brain injury

A diagnosis is made: a severe closed brain injury, the result of falling down the cliff and striking your head. A large hematoma must be surgically removed from the left frontal lobe. Possible frontal, temporal, and diffuse damage. The prescription? Acute care for several weeks. Transfer to a rehabilitation hospital when condition is no longer acute. Probable deficits include short-term memory loss, paralysis of the right side, perception and comprehension problems, possible loss of executive functions, and disinhibition. Long-term outlook: guarded if patient awakens after surgery and shows steady improvement.

This is only a scenario, but it could happen. In fact, it did happen to several patients at HealthSouth RIOSA. Their conditions are currently stable, and both husbands and wives are in continual touch with their case managers. They now understand the program, the procedures, and the chances of recovery. They are involved with every aspect of their spouses' rehabilitation. They are members of the interdisciplinary team.

Right now, you might have a case manager working with you at a particular rehabilitation hospital. You might understand exactly what is going on with your brain-injured loved one. But if you are still overwhelmed by the day-to-day rehabilitation routines, if you cannot comprehend how each therapy works, then read on. We will be your case-manager guides, showing you rehabilitation in action and how the various therapies work toward a common goal: helping the brain-injured patient achieve independence and live life to the fullest potential.

ACUTE DISTRESS

In an ideal world, rehabilitation starts in the emergency room as you are wheeled in, possibly unconscious or confused, after your accident. A neurological team performs a wide range of diagnostic tests, including a blood workup, CT scans, MRIs, and sensory-motor exams; you will be classified according to the Glasgow Coma Scale, which helps determine the severity of your injury and the deficits you are most likely to encounter as you progress. The neurologic team also determines if there is any swelling, fluid buildup, and resulting intracranial pressure, as well as any of the other secondary physical symptoms we described in Chapter Six.

At this point, rehabilitation consists of proper positioning and movement to prevent bed sores, weakened muscles, or spasticity. Sensory stimulation — conversation, soft music, or touching — might be enacted. Vital signs are watched carefully. Respiratory therapists may help you breathe with a ventilator; they will help you cough to clear your lungs and avoid the risk of pneumonia.

At HealthSouth RIOSA we have what is called a "High Observation Unit." Patients can be brought into this unit much earlier than in many rehabilitation hospitals. Here, the patient is dressed every day — shoes, shirt, socks — even if he can't lift his head or move his body. His hair is washed and groomed. Vital signs and life support systems are, of course, constantly monitored, but in addition, routines are established: speech, occupational, and physical therapy is begun. As a nurse in this unit told *Progress Report* magazine, "We begin our work with patients early in the process of recovery, before skills deteriorate even further."

Eventually, the patient's condition stabilizes. Surgery

has been performed. His brain is healing; pressure is down. He is in a confused, agitated state and ripe for more complex rehabilitation. He is transferred from the "High Observation Unit" to a regular room, or from an intensive care unit to a rehabilitation hospital.

REHAB AT WORK

We confess: We're not magicians. Nor are we miracle workers, rainmakers, or alchemists who make gold out of stone. But we are experienced professionals who like what we do. We are professionals, helping patients compensate for deficits and live to their fullest potential. We are educators, teaching families how to cope with a brain-injured loved one. We are knowledgeable and responsible, and we can help a brain-injured patient and his family more than any traditional hospital, emergency ward, or nursing home can.

With all our knowledge, research, and ability, we don't know all the mechanisms of why rehabilitation works, but

---

HEADLINERS

Sometimes emergence from a coma may be assisted by a tug at the emotional heartstrings — at least that's what John P. LaRue, M.S., discovered when he invented a storybook cassette player that a 2-year-old could control with a nudge. For one particular 2-year-old, the cassette played a bedtime story read by his parents. The child eventually understood stimulus-response connection between nudging the cassette into action and hearing his parents read a story, a crucial first step as he came out of his coma.

we do know that it does. We can't always measure in exact terms what happens with a brain-injured patient. In fact, during the first six months after an injury, rapid spontaneous recovery can occur. This natural healing might take place for over two years after the injury. There may be no rhyme or reason, no predictable day of the month when one patient gets his memory back, when another patient begins to understand what she reads, when a third patient stops seeing double.

In actuality, we know a great deal more about why rehabilitation increases the chances for recovery — which is why we've felt a need for this new edition of *Living with Brain Injury*.

No, we can't make spontaneous recovery happen. Nor can we bring dead nerve cells back to life. But what we can do is:

1. Evaluate a patient's needs and establish his goals. In traditional medicine, taking down a medical history and performing a physical exam may be enough to determine a diagnosis and treatment plan. But, as you saw in Chapter Ten, rehabilitation uses the team approach, which can mean up to 12 different staff members, therapists, physicians, and psychologists, who will meet with the patient and his family and analyze his condition. Everyone has a chance to discuss their evaluations and a plan is made — a well-informed and well-thought-out rehabilitation program that takes into account the patient's individual needs, potential, and future goals. This process is also dynamic. It is flexible and ready to be changed when the patient's condition changes.

2. Prevent medical complications. Even the comatose, severely brain-injured patient can benefit from rehabilitation focusing on nutrition, skin care, bladder and bowel care, and prevention of muscle breakdown. Without proper care, a patient can deteriorate and never reach his full potential.

3. Teach a patient compensatory strategies to make up for his disability. A patient may be left with weakness in an arm or difficulty thinking. We can teach strategies to compensate for these and other disabilities.

4. Put the brain's natural healing mechanisms to work to make rehabilitation more efficient and more effective. The brain's ability to compensate for a brain injury is called neural plasticity; it literally finds new pathways to get messages to and from the brain. Therapies, such as constraint therapy, may help accelerate this process. *(You'll be reading all about these exciting new advances in brain injury rehabilitation in Chapter Twelve.)*

5. Maximize those abilities that do start to come back. It's true that many patients might not be able to use their legs again. They might remain paralyzed from the waist down. They might never be able to pronounce words coherently. They might never be able to keep organizational responsibilities straight. But if memory starts to come back, it can be used to help organize thoughts. If problem-solving skills start to return, they can be used to help the patient cope with getting around in a wheelchair.

This kind of rehabilitation is, in the truest sense, a matter of accentuating the positive.

And we do see positive results. We know that we make an impact, because many patients do get better. Some get jobs. They can be independent at home with a minimum amount of supervision.

It makes sense. We keep patients safe in a structured, secure environment. We are consistent in our methods. We teach awareness. We repeat our lessons over and over again, as often as it takes. And, above all, we emphasize *function* above theory or psychology. Helping a brain-injured patient, say, get to a bank, sign a check, and deposit it will do more for his self-confidence, self-esteem, and functional abilities than all the tests, mazes, fill-in-the-blanks, and therapeutic analysis in the world.

But along with consistency, function, repetition, and structure, there are methods to our "madness," the actual techniques used in rehabilitation. Let's briefly review them now and see how they work.

MIND OVER MATTER, OR COGNITIVE REHABILITATION

Knowing isn't necessarily thinking. Cognitive rehabilitation isn't just involved with memory function, executive function, problem-solving skills, and comprehension. It also deals with attention and concentration, appropriate behavior and social communication, activities of daily living, and functioning in the real world — all to the best of a brain-injured person's ability. In fact, knowing is a broad term, involving all the disciplines of rehabilitation. As rehabilitation pioneers Drs. George Prigatano and Yehuda Ben-Yishay define it in

"Cognitive Remediation," their article in *Rehabilitation of the Adult and Child Brain with Traumatic Brain Injury,* cognitive rehabilitation is "the amelioration of the deficits in problem-solving abilities in order to improve functional competence in everyday life situations."

Here's an example of cognitive rehabilitation in action:

After his accident, 15-year-old Charlie couldn't read. After extensive testing, our team agreed that his primary problem was paying attention. He couldn't stay focused on the task at hand.

In fact, Charlie's attention span was so limited that Beth, his speech therapist, could only work with him in five-minute increments. She might have booked 45 minutes a day for therapy, but half of those minutes would be "break time." She'd bring him back into focus by various cognitive remediation techniques, including:

• *Cueing.* If they were working with a workbook and Charlie became distracted, Beth would cue him back to the appropriate point. Other cueing methods include wrist watches with alarm systems set to go off in 10-minute increments and big, brightly colored signs stating, "Time to pay attention!"

• *Strategy teaching.* In the best of all possible rehabilitation worlds, the patient and the therapists work together to come up with strategies to cope with the patient's limitations. In Charlie's case, he and Beth listened to "Books on Tape" in five-minute intervals; they'd then read those same sections in a book. Every five minutes, Charlie's alarm clock would ring, reminding him to pay attention. And every half-hour, he'd take a break. He and Beth would chat about the books he used to read, his war heroes, even the latest movies. After 10 minutes, they'd go back to the task at hand, again setting Charlie's watch for five-minute intervals.

Eventually, Charlie's attention span grew. He no longer needed to be reminded every five minutes to stay focused. Nor would he need long breaks. His problem-solving skills got better, his memory improved, and he was able to read and understand large-print books. And, as an added plus, Charlie also improved his social skills — he was able to discuss books, movies, and life at large with anyone who asked.

• *Altering the environment.* Whenever Beth or anybody else worked with Charlie, they did so in quiet, distraction-free rooms with subdued lighting. The fewer distractions, the fewer stimuli that could tear Charlie's attention away.

• *Overlearning.* New information is "packaged" in what scientists call engrams. These engrams are stored in the brain, ready to be "opened" at a memory cue. But brain-injured patients with memory problems need to create new engrams, or at least new pathways to "unlock" them from storage. Using repetition, patience, consistency structure, and simple explanations, a therapist will teach something over and over again until it has become an engram.

Reading one particular children's book out loud to Charlie over and over again made him finally remember it. When he read the book to himself, he continued to remember. Words began to make sense. What he "overlearned," he carried over to other books. His attention was getting better, his concentration was focused because he now understood what he was reading, and he enjoyed it.

• *Chain of events.* We don't even think about such automatic routines as, say brushing our teeth or putting the water on to boil for coffee. But for someone with a cognitive deficit, each step must be spelled out in sequence. Listen to the 12 steps needed simply to make a peanut butter and jelly sandwich to have with a glass of milk (taken from a HealthSouth RIOSA orientation booklet).

1. Must find peanut butter and jelly on shelf of refrigerator and move them to the counter.
2. Must get a knife out.
3. Must get a loaf of bread out of the pantry.
4. Must get a plate and glass out of the cupboard.
5. Must get milk out of the refrigerator.
6. Must get a napkin out.
7. Must put peanut butter on bread.
8. Must put jelly on bread.
9. Must put two pieces of bread together.
10. Must put milk in the glass.
11. Must put peanut butter and jelly and milk into refrigerator.
12. When finished eating must put dishes in the sink.

In addition to writing these steps down, a therapist will recite them out loud to cue the patient, acting as a "stage manager," watching the patient cope with each step. The therapist also has to make sure that counters and cabinets aren't cluttered, that food items have easy-to-read labeling, that the patient knows how to scan from left to right, top to bottom, to locate the items needed. It's no wonder that brain-injured survivors can become frustrated and depressed! Simple chores and tasks have become elaborate productions.

Unfortunately, even if a brain-injured survivor finally learns how to make a peanut butter and jelly sandwich or how to brush his teeth, chances are he'll forget some of what he learned when he gets back home. Why? Because the structure, quiet, and consistency of the rehabilitation hospital is gone. There are many more distractions, plus the added stress of trying to "make it" in the real world.

But a solution is on its way.

SAT SCORES

SAT stands for Skills Acquisition Training. The term was coined by Norman Namerow, a neurologist specializing in rehabilitation. It aptly described our functional approach to brain injury rehabilitation.

SAT is a total program, involving every member of the team, all of them joined together to retrain a person to function in the real world. Rather than teach someone, say, problem-solving skills on a computer or sequencing with numbered cards, therapists get the patients out in the world, doing what they'll be doing when they re-enter the community. Riding a bus. Reading a map. Going to the supermarket. Answering the phone. Learning functional skills.

The first order of SAT business is to discover the patient's strengths and weaknesses. Does he know how to act in public? Does he shout out rude remarks? Does he get confused? The weak areas are worked on, and the patient's strengths are used to build up his confidence and self-esteem. And, all the while, cognitive functions are being tapped.

When Charlie went out into the community, he became aware of his cognitive limitations in a way he'd never been able to in the hospital. He didn't know how to read a map to get to the library. He couldn't order lunch from a menu. But he was able to discuss books with the librarian when he and his group finally made it to the building. Because he could see both his problems and the positive results of his therapy in real, concrete terms, Charlie became motivated to keep going. Thanks to this functional approach, Charlie continues to improve.

And speaking of motivation, there's another area of therapy that is as important as cognitive rehabilitation. In fact, therapists consider it number one...

HEADLINERS

TAKE ME FOR A RIDE IN YOUR CAR, CAR

Some memories are so deep, so ingrained, and so overused in the past, that brain damage will not destroy them. These "packets of information," or engrams (see "Overlearning," page 138) include singing the words to "Happy Birthday," a short prayer, a multiplication table — even driving a car.

It's not uncommon for many brain-injured people to appear to be able to drive a car. Automatic and overlearned responses may suffice under "ideal" driving conditions. However, problems with reaction time, judgment, and safety awareness can make "real life" driving highly dangerous.

I AM I, AND YOU ARE YOU, OR SELF-AWARENESS TRAINING

It's a reality we're all familiar with: If we deny we have a problem, we never solve it. If we don't feel motivated, we never get out of bed. A brain-injured survivor is no exception. She must get beyond her denial. She must be motivated to reach her potential. She must discover for herself what must be changed and how it can be changed if she is to function in the real world. Each therapy, from individual counseling to social skills training, from speech and language therapy to behavior management, is designed to help a patient reach this goal. Here's an example of self-awareness training in action from our HealthSouth RIOSA files.

A woman in her early 40s had sustained a severe brain injury. She had major muscular problems in her left arm and leg. During her daily physical therapy hour, she tried to do what the therapist asked her to do, with little or no enthusiasm. But during one particular walking session, she had the sense that her arm and leg "clicked" into place, that her whole body, right and left sides, were bearing her weight. She began to relax and there was a clear change in her face. The therapist could see that the woman had suddenly recognized an old muscular "feeling," a sense of comfort that had been lost for a long time. This profound awareness and its subsequent joy was a strong motivation to continue her rehabilitation. In fact, after this self-awareness awakening, she began to make considerable progress.

One of the techniques we have used to teach self-awareness is what we call "the training apartment." Off to the side in our gym, we've placed a sink, an oven, a refrigerator, and cabinets. A private bath. A bed and a table and chairs. When a patient tells us that he doesn't need to be in a rehab hospital, that there's nothing wrong with him, that if he could just go home everything would be fine, we say: "Well. Why don't we spend some time in the "apartment"? I will stay with you, but I want you to show me that you can do everything on your own. If you do well, we will send you home..."

The patient usually doesn't do well. Hopefully, he sees, firsthand, that he can't cook or shower or make the bed. He can no longer deny his problem; he has seen his deficits in action. Although this self-awareness can lead to depression, it usually won't last long. Combined with his busy routine and the support and praise of our staff, his new "self-awareness" will eventually give him the "push" he needs to learn how to live in his brave, new world.

ACTIONS SPEAK LOUDER THAN WORDS, OR BEHAVIOR MANAGEMENT

Pretend we're your former employers and you're a brain-injured patient wanting your old job back. Well, sure, we'll tolerate it if you're slow. We'll even tolerate you if you're not that smart. But we won't put out the welcome mat if you're argumentative, nasty, bossy, and difficult to deal with.

In other words, the biggest roadblock to independent living in society is not the physical deficits involved in brain injury. It's not even the cognitive problems. It's behavior with a capital B.

We weren't the first ones to notice this. One study followed 44 young brain-injured adults for two years after their injuries. Though they had problems with family life, leisure time, and employment, most of the patients were able to adapt to their new situations with one exception: They had lost their old friends because their behavior had changed so much.

But there is hope. Rehabilitation is a learning process, and behavior, too, can be learned, and, even more importantly, relearned. A study of brain-injured patients of all ages, from adolescence to adulthood, by Dr. William Burke and his associates at the New Mexico Highwatch Rehabilitation Center, showed this dramatically The one element each person in this study had in common was the fact that they had each been considered unmanageable by other rehabilitation centers. Six months after participating in a highly structured behavioral management program, 95% of the patients were able to re-enter the community. On an even more promising note, 80% of these same people continued to live independent, responsible lives one year later.

Here are some examples of how behavioral management can work:

• *Correcting problem behavior.* Tim was a model patient. He always came to his therapy appointment on time; he always tried to stay well groomed. But he had one big problem: He would have outrageous outbursts, and would occasionally make some dangerous threats. Ignoring them made it worse. So did anger. Only when the rehabilitation nurse carefully and calmly redirected him did Tim stop his outbursts.

• *Using a reward system.* At HealthSouth RIOSA, we use poker chips as rewards. Here's how it works: When a patient acts in socially appropriate ways during an activity, she gets a certain number of chips which can be cashed in for rewards. A reward might be an extra hour of television at night, or a field trip. But when the patient has an aggressive outburst, she simply doesn't get any chips for that session, and, consequently, no reward. We never punish and take away chips. We reward appropriate behavior.

• *Implementing self-monitoring techniques.* It's exactly what it sounds like: Self-monitoring helps patients learn appropriate behavior by thinking before acting out. Billy used a daily log to keep tabs on his behavior. The log was divided into two columns: "Appropriate Behavior" and "Inappropriate Behavior." Billy would put an "x" in the column that applied after each therapy session. He also received his chips when he had three or more x's in the "Appropriate Behavior" column.

• *Utilizing negotiation.* Joan's therapist told her that if she just sticks to wheelchair practice for 10 minutes, she'll get an extra chip.

• *Participating in support groups.* "Nobody understands"... "I feel all alone"... "I wish there was someone I could talk to..." There's power in numbers, especially when the ranks are made up of people in the same situation as you. They can offer true empathy, understanding, and hope. Guided by therapists, brain-injured patients get a chance to communicate with others in this group format. For the first time, they get to express their thoughts and feelings to people who have been there. Communication skills, social skills training, language skills, self-awareness — all these are developed within the group format. Support groups can involve everything from substance abuse problems to surviving in the world.

Behavior management permeates every aspect of the rehabilitation program. It's a useful approach no matter what the therapy. A patient gets a chip for a job well done. An occupational therapist calmly corrects the behavior of a rude teen. A physical therapist negotiates — and gets — an extra 15 minutes to work on her patient's gait.

The results permeate the entire therapy program. If a patient feels better about himself, more confident and calm, he'll be more motivated to practice his cognitive skills. If he's getting along with others, he is less likely to act selfishly or throw a childish tantrum in front of his new friends.

Cognitive skills and behavior. Feelings and thoughts. You now know the basic elements behind a good rehabilitation program. Let's take a few moments to look again at what the other therapies work to accomplish:

"SPEAK EASY": SPEECH AND LANGUAGE THERAPY

You will find the speech-language therapist doing more than what her title might imply. She also teaches eating and swallowing techniques, and focuses on cognitive and communication skills — for instance, teaching a patient with verbal expression problems to use gestures or writing to help communicate his thoughts and needs. She will construct a "memory book" to help him keep track of what has gone on during the day The memory book might include snapshots of family members, pets, and hospital staff, and brief notes made by a therapist or by the patient himself after a specific activity. It may also include:

- A calendar to help him recall the day and date.
- Sequencing instructions for various activities.
- Large-printed cues, to use a knife and fork, for instance, or, in Charlie's case, to pay more attention.

Speech and language therapy also involves the patient's family. Learning to read a paragraph is one thing, but a relative might want her loved one to be able to read his prescription or write down phone messages. A good therapist will concentrate on these particular, practical skills. One patient at HealthSouth RIOSA had little use of her hands. She had memory deficits and permanent speech damage. But she and her speech therapist were able to work out a communication technique. The patient would point out letters on a chart, spelling out words she wanted to say. The first time she was told that there was a chance she could communicate in the world, the patient spelled out her first message: "Please help me."

LEARNING BY DOING, OR OCCUPATIONAL THERAPY

During her occupational therapy hour, you'll find your loved one working on her safety awareness, her perceptual problems, her executive functions. But, while all these skill trainings are going on, the underlying object is to help her perform functional tasks. She might not see her blouse the way you see it; she might try to put her head through a sleeve. She might try to comb her hair with a toothbrush. Through occupational therapy sessions, she will not only learn how to button her blouse, but the sequencing order

---

HEADLINERS

MEMORY BOOK ENTRIES

(NOTE: These are actual entries written by therapists after a session. Patients with memory loss problems will read through them later.)

7:50 a.m.: Lucy, I came in and we got you dressed. I helped you with your breakfast. Dr. Senelick came in. You spoke with him and showed him your fingernails. You watched TV. You're doing great. We love you. – Peggy

8:30 a.m.: Now you are sitting up in your chair making short work of your breakfast. There is absolutely nothing wrong with your appetite! – Nell

1:00-1:30 p.m.: Speech with Judy. You invited me to your party. We talked about what we would do at your party. We played the "Imagining" Game. You did well and earned 2 chips.

---

for getting dressed.

Occupational therapists work on other activities of daily living such as grooming, bathing, and hygiene. If there is arm or hand weakness or a lack of coordination, the therapist will work on upper-extremity exercises, perhaps using a splint or brace to decrease spasticity or increase upper extremity function.

LIFE IN THE REAL WORLD

At HealthSouth, on any given day, you might get a whiff of a class' home-baked chocolate chip cookies fresh from the oven. You might notice the freshly seeded vegetable and flower gardens outside. You might see a group of brain-injured patients clutching paper bags filled with groceries coming back from a visit to the supermarket. Or they could be bringing souvenirs from a field trip to a nearby museum. You might overhear a patient pretending to call a prospective boss on a "fake" phone, learning what to say and how to say it. You might walk past a room where people are discussing the newest and latest computer microchip. You might see a group barbecuing burgers on an outside grill or playing volleyball in an open field. As you can see, activities of daily living (ADLs) are not just "tasks." They can actually be fun! But these ADLs do have a serious objective: teaching independence.

Recreational therapy. Music and art therapy. Vocational therapy. Budgeting classes. Social skills training. All these are designed to make the brain-injured patients re-entry into the community as smooth and stress-free as possible.

LET'S GET PHYSICAL, OR PHYSICAL THERAPY

Physical therapy is as much a part of the treatment package as anything else. Cognitive, behavioral, and self-awareness training are taught as patients learn how to transfer themselves from a wheelchair to a bed, from a sitting position to standing.

Physical therapy sessions also concentrate on range-of-motion exercises. As a result of their injury, many patients suffer from spasticity, or a prolonged contraction of the mus-

HEADLINERS

A DAY IN THE LIFE*

Charles S.: Moderate Brain-Injured 15-year-old Patient

7:15-7:45	Breakfast with other patients and staff
7:45-8:30	Activities of Daily Living (ADL) training (encompassing Occupational Therapy)
8:30-9:00	Current Events group (encompassing Occupational Therapy and Speech Therapy)
9:00-9:30	Wheelchair Mobility Group (Physical Therapy)
9:30-10:30	Speech Therapy
10:30-11:00	Occupational Therapy
11:00-12:00	Physical Therapy
12:00-12:30	Lunch
12:30-1:00	Rest
1:00-1:30	Rehabilitation Counseling (Individual Therapy)
1:30-2:00	Occupational Therapy
2:00-3:00	Social Skills Training (Encompassing Speech)
3:00-3:30	Rest
3:30-5:00	Community Reorientation Outing (Recreational Therapy)
5:00-5:30	Nursing (Physical Therapy and ADL)
6:00-7:30	Rest
7:30-8:00	Survivors Support Group

*This is meant only as an example of various activities. Most days would not involve all of these activities.

cles caused by disinhibition similar to the one that triggers socially inappropriate behavior. The physical therapist teaches patients how to relax and loosen these tight muscles.

Specific exercises can strengthen weakened muscles and increase overall endurance. Illness and inactivity dramatically reduce a person's endurance, making it difficult to get through the day without frequent rest periods. Once strength is adequate, it's possible to progress to walking. Initially, a patient may walk only between parallel bars and require a good deal of help from the therapist. Over time, he will graduate to a walker or a cane with four legs (quad cane), and hopefully on to independent walking.

A SPOONFUL OF MEDICINE, OR PSYCHOPHARMACOLOGY

Remember this slogan: *The best medicine is frequently no medicine at all.*

Drugs can cloud already foggy minds. They can slow down the thinking process. They can cause damaging side effects. But if a patient is severely depressed or suicidal, if he has seizures, if his attention deficits or agitation border on the dangerous, that's a different story. Medicine that works on the chemical imbalances in the brain may be necessary. Very briefly, here's a rundown of the medications commonly used in brain-injury rehabilitation:

• *Antipsychotics.* These drugs work on the neurotransmitter called dopamine, stopping it from stimulating a dopamine receptor in the next nerve cell. These drugs have been used for schizophrenia for years. In brain-injured patients, they effectively stop agitation, hyperactivity, hallucinations, and hostility. Unfortunately, while these drugs stop inappropriate behavior, they also cause memory, learning, and cognitive problems. They also have side effects, including movement disorders. Although newer medications have fewer side effects, they should still be used sparingly and for as short a time as possible. They should also be avoided immediately following the injury because they may contribute to further neurological injury. *Common brand names: Haldol®, Prolixin®, Resperidal®, and Zyprexa®.*

• *Beta Blockers.* These drugs are most commonly used for high blood pressure, migraines, and heart problems. They get their name by effectively "blocking" the beta-adrenergic receptors in the forebrain that carry the messages for anxiety, nervousness, and sweating. Because they block debilitating emotions, they may be used by musicians, actors, and other performers before going onstage. In brain injuries they are used to treat agitation, aggression, and violence. Side effects include dizziness, apathy, depression, impotence, and nightmares. *Common names: Inderal® and Corgard®.*

• *Psychostimulants.* These are mainly used for hyperactive children. But because they work on inattention, distraction, disorganization, impulsivity, mood swings, fatigue, and apathy, they're frequently given to brain-injured patients. Psychostimulants increase the levels of the brain chemical dopamine, an inhibitory neurotransmitter. There is some experimental evidence to suggest they help the healing of brain cells. Their side effects include insomnia, anorexia, headaches, and irritability. *Common brand names: Ritalin®, Provigil® and Cylert®.*

• *Lithium.* Believe it or not, this drug was first discovered in spas in ancient Greece; it was recognized early on as a stabilizing force. Lithium is commonly used for treating manic-depressive illnesses. In brain-injured patients, it's used to stop aggressive behavior and instability. But it must be closely monitored; too much lithium can become toxic. Side effects include diarrhea, tremors, and, at toxic levels, confusion and disorientation. *Common names: Lithium Carbonate and Lithobid®.*

• *Dopaminergic Agents.* These drugs also work on the dopamine receptors at the synapses of the brain; they are used primarily in comatose and low-level patients in an attempt to shorten coma and improve functioning. Side effects include dizziness, nausea, and confusion. *Common names: Parlodel® and Amantadine®.*

• *Anticonvulsants.* If a brain-injured person suffers from seizures, these drugs can control them. They may also stop episodic explosive behavior, but primarily in patients with abnormal brain wave tests. Side effects include dizziness and sedation. *Common names: Dilantin®, Tegretol®, and Depakote®.*

• *Antidepressants.* A depressed patient might be given an antidepressant to help improve the brain's chemistry The new generation of antidepressants, SSRIs, work on a chemical called serotonin. They can have a dramatic effect on feelings of despair or hopelessness in a short period of time. *Side effects include insomnia, restlessness, or impotence. Common brand names: Prozac®, Zoloft®, Paxil®, and Effexor®.*

In this chapter we've examined the many different types of therapy that are important to a patient's recovery. There remains, however, one more important area to discuss: the new exciting area of neural plasticity.

CHAPTER TWELVE

NEURAL PLASTICITY: THE EXCITING NEW FUTURE OF RECOVERY

"After several months of rehab, I found that my speech had improved to the point where I was having conversations almost as easily as before my accident. My doctor told me that my brain had actually rewired itself. Thanks to a new form of functional therapy, my brain was receiving and sending messages in new routes, like a highway detour, while it took care of the repairs."

A 24-year-old woman and HealthSouth outpatient who had suffered a brain injury in a car accident

Approximately five years ago, in a laboratory at the University of Texas in Houston, Dr. Randolph J. Nudo and a group of monkeys began to make history. It began with a series of experiments in which the monkeys, paralyzed in one hand, were separated into three distinct groups.

One group received good care, food and water, and a clean cage. But they received no rehabilitation, no therapy to get their hand moving again.

The second group not only received quality care, but some basic therapy. They were taught how to move their arm, but were not given any exercises for individual finger movements or to perform any functional tasks, such as picking up a ball and throwing it, waving hello, or scratching their face. They didn't show any more improvement than the group who received no therapy at all. In other words, rudimentary therapy was as good as, well, nothing.

But the third group of monkeys was a different story. They received the top of the line "monkey rehab." They not only received the quality care of the first two groups, but they were also put to work: they were required to perform specific tasks that utilized individual fingers to pick and grab food pellets from small wells. And this group? *They did substantially better than the other two groups — and they had much more success in the return of the function of the paralyzed hand.*

This alone would show that the quality of rehabilitation is more important than the rehabilitation itself. But there's more:

When Dr. Nudo did sophisticated electrical stimulation studies on this last group of monkeys, they revealed something that was not seen in the other two groups. The area of the brain next to the damaged area was the place where shoulder movement was normally controlled. But now, in this third group of monkeys, this "shoulder movement locale" had increased in size — and had taken over the function of the hand.

In other words, the area of the brain that had been damaged (in this case the part that controlled hand movement) could no longer function and a different area of the brain took over the job.

The brain had literally rerouted its messages, transporting messengers away from the usual neurotransmitters and sending them down a different passageway — with ultimately the same result. In the same way a superhighway will change the course of the way a car will get from one town to another, the brain will change the way the message gets to where it needs to go.

But it gets there just the same.

Dr. Randolph J. Nudo and his monkeys had proved the rewiring of the brain, an exciting new aspect for brain injury rehabilitation, offering new hope and new treatment options for those people who thought they might not be able to function at the same capacity as before.

Neural plasticity was born.

BUT FIRST...

Although Dr. Nudo and his colleagues provided proof for the theory of neural plasticity, the idea of a flexible, resilient brain was formulated long before plastic was even a word in our dictionary.

In 1915, physician Shepherd Ivory Franz observed that many motor disabilities in people who had come to his hospital seemed to have occurred after the accident or stroke. In other words, the paralysis of a hand or a finger or a leg seemed to happen from a lack of use, not from an accident-induced inability. He called this phenomenon "uncared for paralysis" and, in 1917, he joined forces with another researcher, Dr. R. Ogden, and discovered that when the affected leg or arm was restrained (forced-use therapy):

- Massaging the unrestrained affected limb showed absolutely no results...
- ...forced use of the restrained leg or arm led to significant recovery.

Working closely with the theory of learned helplessness, Psychologist Martin Seligmann found that animals who failed to obtain positive feedback for their efforts eventually "gave up" — or learned helplessness. They just stopped trying.

Years later, in 1980, Dr. Edward Taub took these findings one step further and discovered that this learned non-use was more destructive to successful rehabilitation than no rehabilitation at all. He began to formulate his theories of constraint therapy in which the paralyzed limb is forced into action.

How does this relate to neural plasticity?

Easy.

Let's go back to our new highway. In order to build that road, pour the concrete, put up the railings, you need to know that cars will be using it. The highway has to be used. Otherwise, it will fall into disrepair from non-use. Weeds will begin to peek out from the concrete; potholes will form; roadside stations will close up shop. The first route might have closed down from a traumatic accident or an "act of God", but the second route will have the same exact fate — if it's not used.

But if cars are forced to use that new highway, directed with arrows and signs and guards to go on this new road, they surely will. Eventually, they'll be humming along, the sun on the windshield, as if they'd always ridden on this road.

Brain plasticity and the new rehabilitation therapy have the exact same principles behind them:

By forcing rehabilitation patients to use the affected arm or leg, the brain is stimulated to reorganize its heady mass of synapses and neurotransmitters. It rewires a new route and literally takes charge: Move that leg! But instead of, say, giving the command in French, it's now saying to do the job in English. Instead of taking Route 23, it's telling the message to take Highway 10.

The job gets done and rehabilitation does its work.

THE GRAY MATTER

Neil had always wanted to try skydiving. It looked so glorious, so free. He was careful, though. An 18-year-old college student, he had his whole future ahead of him; he had plans to be a doctor and didn't want to take too many risks.

But the call of the sky kept taunting him. When his new girlfriend decided to join him in his skydiving passion, he figured why not. Thousands of people try it; thousands of people come away unscathed.

They went about it methodically, filled with common sense, taking lessons, getting fit. Neil's first skydive went perfectly; he jumped out of the plane, the engines roaring. He floated for a moment, then began to drop; he felt like he was flying through the clouds. He pulled out his parachute and it was like a miracle: he began to gently float down to the earth.

Neil was delirious; he had never felt so free, so exuberant, in his life. Unfortunately, his landing didn't prove as heavenly as his flight. Neil accidentally hit his head on a rock as gravity pulled him down to earth. Lucky for him, his spinal cord was uninjured; the same could not be said of his brain. Neil suffered a brain injury on the right side of his head and after a two-week stay at a hospital's trauma division, he was sent to a rehabilitation center.

The prognosis looked good. Neil was young and in good shape; he had had bruising (a contusion) of his brain, but the swelling had gone down with no after-effects. He had not gone into a coma in the hospital; he had been in shock and had blacked out, but it lasted only a few minutes.

However, Neil was left with a slight paralysis (hemiparesis) on the left side of his body. He couldn't use his left hand too well and he could barely use his left leg.

But with proper therapy, his rehabilitation team was confident that he would be fine. He might even be able to go back to medical school some day.

One of the new therapies the rehab team wanted to try

> *"It is not only the kind of head injury*
> *that matters, but the kind of head."*
> *– Symonds*

on Neil was constraint therapy. His unaffected right arm was put in a mitten, starting at 16 hours each day. He couldn't use his unaffected arm for anything — and he was forced to use his weak right arm to brush his teeth, eat, dress, you name it.

Neil also used weight-supported treadmill training (WSTT) — a new and somewhat controversial therapy. He was put in a harness over a treadmill that was moving at a very slow speed. He walked — and was forced to use his weaker right leg. Because the walking motion stimulates the actual gait patterns that are used in unassisted walking, the theory goes that it also stimulates the brain into creating new passageways to get the bad leg moving again. It seemed to work for Neil; he was walking better, stronger, after a few weeks of WSTT.

But, needless to say, it was slow going for Neil. However, he continues to make excellent progress. Six months after his accident, Neil is seeing his rehabilitation therapist on an outpatient basis. He no longer keeps his right arm in a mitten and he no longer has to "fight his brain" to use his left arm. His left arm is almost functioning as well as his right now; his brain has marked a new highway to left arm movement and motor coordination; it was stimulated to do so by being forced to send messages to and from the damaged arm. Neil's progress is proof of the theories of neural plasticity and learned non-use.

PLASTIC MOLDS

Like anything else in life, neural plasticity is not a perfect science. The jury is still out on constraint therapy and weight-supported treadmills. There are numerous variables that must be taken into account in order for this new rehabilitation to have the highest success rate:

Timing is Everything

Think of a telephone cable network, a series of wires connecting one to the other, all interrelated and all connected to a main source. In many ways, the brain and its passageways are like a series of wires going this way and that way, all interconnected and coded by color. When you have a brain injury, things stop. The connections between wires are immediately lost. Messages cannot get through. In order for the wires to reconnect, for instructions on, say, moving a hand, remembering a name, buttoning a blouse, to be understood and enacted, rehabilitation must start as soon as possible. When your phone goes out, it needs to be fixed yesterday. The same goes with your brain. The sooner rehab begins, the less time there is for the "dust to settle" and the connection to be lost forever.

A Wounded State

We've already seen how the location of a brain injury is crucial to determining successful recovery after a brain injury. But neural plasticity theories show that the location in the brain is not always as important as the location of the lesion in the neural network. In other words, if the brain injury occurred on a crucial highway in the brain, even if it was, say, far from the king of executive function, the frontal cerebral cortex, the brain injury would be serious. Messages would not be able to connect easily; network roads would not be able to connect.

And if that lesion were not only a roadblock on an important highway, but a big, traffic-stopping one, the success rate for recovery would be seriously low indeed.

The good news is that plasticity, by its very definition, means molding, growth, flexibility. Paths regenerate on their own; networks start up nearby; function returns on a different highway with proper rehabilitation as lesions heal.

Sci-fi Thriller

Before the birds and the bees, there were sperm cells and egg cells. Those cells grew and developed into human beings, all of us with brains and hearts and lungs and limbs. Early on in this developmental process, we grow stem cells that, when turned on by certain growth factors, will turn into specific parts of our body. Scientists have actually learned how to harvest these stem cells and grow them, like tomatoes or roses, into brain cells, motor neurons, or spinal cord cells. When these new cells have been injected into the brains of animals in laboratory settings, the animals not only survive, but some of the deficits caused by injury have healed. The nerve growth research has only just begun, but it holds much exciting promise for treating brain injury and paralysis.

You Don't Eat These Sprouts

Think about your garden — or a garden you've seen on television. When you cut a bush or plant back to prune it, the plant grows back bigger, more lush, and healthier; it literally sprouts beautiful new growth. After a brain injury, the wires in your brain, those axons and dendrites of a nerve cell, start sprouting new "stems," new growth to seek out new connections. This is called collateral sprouting, and this regeneration is an important element of neural plasticity. With good rehabilitation, those new stems can be trained to connect the correct way and traffic in the brain can hum along as it did before...

Learning New Things Every Day

When Dr. Nudo did his groundbreaking research with his monkeys, he discovered that it wasn't enough to retrain them to use their hands. As he said, "Changes in the motor cortex are driven by acquisition of new motor skills and not simply by motor use." In other words, it's not enough to have the monkeys tapping their fingers; he wanted them to learn to pick out food pellets from a well; he wanted them to learn to think, to figure out how to use their hands to get what they wanted.

This is true with rehabilitation in humans as well. It isn't enough for you to use your weakened limb in physical therapy. You also have to do specific tasks, such as getting dressed or writing a note. By forcing your affected arm to work at different tasks, your brain becomes stimulated; the whole network surrounding the damaged area becomes active; highway branches (synapses and dendrites) sprout up; other areas of the brain pick up the functional slack.

Neural plasticity is an exciting new area of research — and the new rehabilitation has only just begun to see results. As with any new therapy, time will tell how precise it really is. Further studies need to be done to determine exactly when constraint therapy needs to begin, and how long it should be applied. Diagnostic tools must become as advanced as the research to know how much to do and when to begin.

But one thing is certain: There is hope and excitement and a new world awaiting only a highway away....

CHAPTER THIRTEEN

THE FAMILY CIRCLE

"He looks like my husband, but
he's not... My husband's gone."
A *wife of a HealthSouth*
brain-injured patient

• Statistics show that between 40% and 50% of all marriages in which one of the spouses has been brain-injured end in divorce, and many professionals in the field put the percentage much higher.

• A study of 200 families in which one member has been brain-injured found that the caregivers felt isolated and trapped. They felt neither married nor single, and their sexual and emotional needs were unfulfilled.

• A study of wives one year after their spouses were brain-injured discovered that they found their husbands selfish, childish, demanding, and dependent.

• The children of brain-injured parents also suffer. Studies found that they are often anxious, irritable, depressed, unruly, and doing poorly in school. Why? As Michael E. Howard, Ph.D., writes: "Children catch it from both ends: They are obviously ignored by the brain-injured patient who is hospitalized, but they are also often ignored by the spouse who is so caught up in his or her own grief."

• Since most brain injuries occur in men, it's mothers who truly must "mother" — sometimes an entire family circle at once.

• Research has found that when someone suffers long-lasting harm from a brain injury, his family's sense of burden increases over time, At six months, relatives felt that their brain-injured loved one's most outstanding problems were loss of affection, poor control of temper, social withdrawal, lack of energy, cruelty, meanness, and unreasonableness. At one year, these same relatives felt just as strongly about these same issues. As more time elapsed, the relatives' capacity for coping with and accepting these problems decreased. A different study discovered that five years after an injury, 74% of relatives still said their brain-injured family member's personality problems were tough to take.

Harsh statistics, but true. It is indeed, as Dr. Robert Sbordone states, the families who "are the real victims of a brain injury." They too need attention and structure. They too need to be educated and trained. They too need nurturing and support. In fact, a good rehabilitation program spends extensive time working with the patients' families.

FAMILY TIES

One of the crucial elements for a good outcome is family support. In fact, Michael E. Howard, Ph.D., found that a key family member, one who is involved in all facets of the treatment plan, offering support, guidance, and help to his brain-injured relative, is the single most important factor for successful rehabilitation.

But whatever your role in the new family dynamics, the best support you can give is educated support. And, in order to be educated and most helpful, you should expect your rehabilitation team to:

• Give *permission* to your family to ask questions, as many as you want, without feeling intimidated.

• Provide information and *more* information about brain injury. The more you know, the better equipped you'll be to handle any problem that comes up.

• Find those key persons in the family who will be a pillar of strength, support, and involvement, but, at the same time, find ways that they can get "time off."

• Assign one person, either a social worker or a case manager, to handle your family's questions or problems — from insurance and financial structures to family therapy referrals — to help you all cope.

• Encourage support groups. Nothing will help a stressed-out and confused family more than a group of sympathetic, understanding peers who have "been there" themselves.

• Involve your entire family in all aspects of rehabilitation, from the confusion and isolation of intensive care through proper help in the activities of daily living.

FAMILY CRIES

A study of over 100 mothers of brain-injured children found that the biggest stressors for them were their child's behavior problems. One mother's complaint was her daughter's dramatic and abrupt mood swings. Another mother complained of her son's sudden bursts of temper that were loud and profane.

The second biggest stressors were family difficulties — the vicissitudes of life that continue even while tragedy strikes: A death in the family, poor sibling adjustment, financial burdens.

Other mothers worried about their child's recovery and the future. One mother feared "the kind of life my son would have if I died, got sick, or emotionally burned out." Slow progress, the very real worry of rehabilitation expenses, all take their toll.

Most of these mothers felt that the most stressful time was right after the accident, while they were waiting to see if their child would live or come out of a coma.

However, there were a significant number of mothers who felt just the opposite. For them, the most nerve-wracking time was after their child returned home. Suddenly, mothers lost their freedom. Their teen-age children could not be left home alone and unattended. They needed constant care which was both exhausting and debilitating to the mothers.

Others mentioned lack of communication between themselves and their child's doctors, and difficulty in finding others who understand what brain injury is all about.

Finally, there was always that sadness over what their child had lost and over the lack of support from one-time friends and from other family members, As one mother whose son had spent time at HealthSouth RIOSA said, "All of us have to face reality. It's like there's this person, then there's the accident, then another person emerges. You have to learn new ways of living. You have to cope with a new life."

You, too, can come out of the trauma intact. Here's some guidance to provide reassurance and to help make your adjustment easier and quicker.

> ### HEADLINERS
>
> *LIKE A NOVEL*
>
> *Ernest Hemingway suffered from a diagnosed depressive disorder and alcoholism. Less well-known was the fact that he had at least five head injuries during his life, one of them the result of a severe airplane crash in Africa. His increasing difficulty in writing, his excessive drinking, his depression, and even his ultimate suicide were possibly rooted in his brain injuries. If only we knew then what we know now about brain injury.*

• *Anger, frustration, and sorrow are natural emotions for close relatives of brain-injured patients.* Yes, it's true. You can grieve. You can feel angry at this person who changed your life. You can feel down in the dumps and even show a sour face to your brain-injured loved one. Family caregivers who feel guilty when they feel angry, who chastise themselves for not being "perfect," will only get depressed, overwhelmed, and sick. After months of taking care of someone who is greedy, angry, childish, and unhappy, it makes absolute sense for you to occasionally say, "Be quiet!"

• *Caregivers must take care of themselves first.* Look at any family rehabilitation booklet. Talk to any case manager or doctor. Before you can give to someone else, you must give to yourself. You must schedule free time. You must have "space." Some of the ways you can be good to yourself are:

- Eat right
- Express your feelings
- Seek professional help for emotional or adjustment problems
- Avoid drug and alcohol abuse
- Be kind to yourself
- Buy yourself a present
- Exercise regularly to relieve stress
- Let others help
- Join a family support group
- Ask questions!!!

- *Trust your instincts.* There will come a time when you must rely on your own conscience and judgment, even if it puts you in conflict with your loved one. Like the child who won't eat his vegetables, your brain-injured loved one might not know what's best for him. Combine his arguments with the well-meaning but contradictory advice other family members inevitably give, and you could remain frozen, unable to do anything, forever. Take charge. Armed with what you've learned, you can handle it.

- *The role changes that inevitably take place are emotionally draining for everyone.* You don't have to pretend that your spouse, the one-time wage earner, responsible partner, and emotional helpmate, makes you happy now that he has turned into a willful, dependent person. Nor do you have to "put on a happy face" when your adult, formerly independent child comes home bedridden and helpless. It's a terrible state of affairs. Roles that have been in place for years, family behaviors that were ingrained for so

HEADLINERS

THE FIRST COPING STRATEGY — AND POSSIBLY THE BEST

Odysseus was a traveler as Homer chronicled in his ancient classic, the Odyssey. *He constantly ran up against disasters and villainous monsters, but always overcame the odds. Odysseus thought up one of his cleverest ruses as his ship was nearing Circe, the bewitching siren of the rocks. If he or his sailors heard Circe's song, they would become hypnotized and crash against the rocks in a horrible death. Rather than pray to the gods or tell his sailors to use self-control, Odysseus simply filled their ears with beeswax, effectively stopping them from hearing the siren's call.*

The moral? Don't always try to make your brain-injured loved one use self-control. Sometime it's just a superhuman task. Instead figure out a way to circumvent the problem.

long they were automatic, family interactions that were once comfortably predictable, are no more. And because these changes occurred so suddenly, there's been no chance to adjust, no time for insights, no thoughts or game plan to help you carry on. Now, more than ever, you need to ask those questions and seek the professional help of your case manager or hospital social worker.

• *There may be little you can do to change your loved one, so there's no need to feel guilty when you see no improve-*

ment. It's true. And, as hard-boiled as this statement is, it's also liberating. It frees you from the shackles of guilt. You can take care of yourself and rejoin the human race.

• *When the welfare of your children is at stake, you must explore your divided loyalties and accurately weigh your responsibilities.* This is a painful issue, one that both families and case managers tend to gloss over. But the fact remains that if brain-injured spouses have become abusive — even though it's through no fault of their own — you might have to figure out other living and caregiving arrangements.

FAMILY BINDS

Muriel D. Lezak, Ph.D., who came up with the above statements families need to hear, has also outlined the six stages families typically go through when a loved one is injured. They are:

STAGE I: OUT OF REACH

Time Since Injury: 1 to 3 months

Family's Perceptions of Their Loved One: He's hurt, weak, tired, and inactive.

Family's Expectation for Their Loved One:
Full recovery by one year.

Family Circle's Reaction: Happy and hopeful.

STAGE II: UP IN THE AIR

Time Since Injury: 1-3 months to 6-9 months, possibly indefinitely

Family's Perceptions of Their Loved One: He's not

cooperating. Not motivated and self-centered.

Family's Expectation for Their Loved One:
Full recovery, if he'll try harder.

Family Circle's Reaction: Bewildered, anxious, and scared.

STAGE III: DOWN AND OUT

Time Since Injury: 6-9 months to 9-24 months — or indefinitely

Family's Perceptions of Their Loved One:
Irresponsible, egocentric, cranky, and lazy!

Family's Expectation for Their Loved One:
Independence — if they only knew how to help him.

Family Circle's Reaction: Discouraged and depressed. Feelings of guilt and "going crazy"

STAGE IV: NO WAY OUT

Time Since Injury: More than 9 months

Family's Perception's of Their Loved One: He's different and difficult to be around. A child.

Family's Expectation of Their Loved One: No hope, but lingering wish for independence that they cannot provide.

Family Circle's Reaction: Despair. A feeling of being "trapped."

STAGE V: PROFOUND SADNESS

Time Since Injury: Over 15 months; usually short-lived

Family's Perception of Their Loved One: He's turned

into a child who is completely dependent.

Family's Expectation for Their Loved One: None.

Family Circle's Reaction: Grief and deep mourning.

STAGE VI: LOST AND FOUND

Time Since Injury: 18 to 24 months — or longer

Family's Perception of Their Loved One: He is and will be a dependent child.

Family's Expectation for Their Loved One: Whatever he can — and wants — to achieve for himself.

Family Circle's Reaction: A dramatic emotional change. Acceptance of what is and "stepping back" from their personal anguish and pain.

Typical, yes. But by no means absolute. Every family is unique, and the way you care for your brain-injured loved one will reflect that individually just as researchers have been able to generalize about the reactions a typical family might face. They've also been able to describe some typical behavior that helps create these negative reactions. Let's go over a few of these "brain teasers" now with some "winning plays" to help you cope:

Brainteaser #1: Overeating

Oh, the joys of food. There's nothing like simmering soup on a winter's day, a refreshing iced drink when it's hot, a fresh baked cake... Unfortunately these simple eating pleasures are much more complicated when it comes to brain-injured patients. Initially, they need to eat to make up for the nourishment they lost when first injured. Later, many caregivers are pleased to see that their patient is eating, especially when he might have spent months being fed in the hospital through a tube. A good appetite is a sign of health. And love, after all, is equated with food.

But this "health" can easily turn into an insatiable appetite, and your patient can get bigger and bigger. Part of the reason may be organic: The hypothalamus, which regulates appetite, may have been damaged from the brain injury. There's an emotional aspect as well, especially if the patient had had weight problems in the past.

WINNING PLAYS: If the problem is organic, seek out professional help. If it's an emotional reaction, remove the food from your kitchen. Offer alternate distractions. Your loved one won't think so much about eating if he's busy swimming, or gardening, or sewing.

Brainteaser #2: Agitation, Outbursts, and Temper Tantrums

Your husband constantly paces his room. Your wife keeps jumping up from her bed. Your son tells you that you're fat and ugly. Your daughter screams curses at the top of her lungs. None of this behavior is unusual. As we have seen in previous chapters, brain injury can cause disinhibition. Emotionally, your loved one will probably be less patient.

He will be confused and troubled. He will be anxious and unable to focus on social skills. It may just be a phase, but be prepared for the possibility that he'll have a more volatile personality for the rest of his life. Fortunately, brain-injured survivors don't always remember their outbursts. A violent temper flare-up is often over quickly; typically it wasn't the result of deep-seated hostility.

WINNING PLAYS: Be calm and structure your routines. Your agitated loved one needs to feel secure. Ignore outbursts, and warn friends and families when they come to call. Redirect your angry loved one to another topic or goal.

Brainteaser #3: Depression

It's very common, but it's not fun. However, take heart. Your loved one's morose behavior, his lack of interest in life, his excessive sleeping — all may be signs of progress. He is no longer denying his deficits, and he has begun the slow road to recovery and acceptance. Some other symptoms include:

- Passivity
- Excessive television watching
- Loss of ability to feel pleasure

WINNING PLAYS: If you feel your loved one is acting suicidal in any way, notify a doctor immediately. Try to divert her — enlist her in a game or a walk in the fresh air. Don't blame yourself. It's not your fault. Continue to be pleasant. Ask your physician about the possible use of anti-depressant medication. Eventually, the depression may lift and make room for acceptance.

Brainteaser #4: Increased or Decreased Sexuality

Sexuality, an uncomfortable topic for discussion even in the best of circumstances, can be particularly painful where brain injury is involved because of all of the corollary

---

HEADLINERS

Sunday, December 3

"When Dad came to get me I came downstairs and fixed my own breakfast (cornflakes - 1 1/2 bowls). Then we watched TV while Daddy was working on a carving of a runner. Mom came down around 10:00. We talked about how many more days until I get to come home to stay. I realized it wasn't that much longer (9 days!). We went upstairs to get dressed and I decided I wanted to put my stamps from Turkey and Germany in my stamp book. I ended up putting 2 of the six packets in the book through the day. About 5:00 Daddy, Colleen, and I went out shopping (Pik & Save) and to pick up some pizza for dinner. I also looked through my photo album and could really see how much I'd improved since I'd had my accident."

— From a memory book entry written by a HealthSouth RIOSA patient with her parents' help to compensate for short-term memory loss. Looking through it later, she would remember her day.

---

problems: possible loss of love, role reversal, and the physical differences in your sexual partner. With brain injury, increased or decreased sexuality is usually a result of damage in the brain. Sexual hyperactivity is a part of disinhibition, the loss of that "civilized" social censor that keeps all of us on a reasonably even keel.

WINNING PLAYS: If your spouse is no longer interested, make sure he's always well-groomed and dressed. If he feels good about himself, he might reassert his sexuality. If he's hyperactive, you probably won't want to go anywhere with him, which can lead to social withdrawal and depression for you both. Instead of hiding, find a support group for him where his behavior can be pointed out. An outpatient rehabilitation program can also be of help. Further, examine your own feelings and needs. Are you afraid sex will further damage your loved one? Are you afraid that the brain injury will prevent you from having children? Remember the adage we mentioned at the beginning of this chapter:

ASK QUESTIONS!!!

Brainteaser #5: Lack of Motivation

It's hard to get going when you are confused, depressed, or overwhelmed. But it's equally hard to listen when the person you love tells you, "I don't want to go to the beach... I don't want to eat dinner... I don't want to help you fold the laundry... I don't want to do anything but lie here on the couch and watch reruns of 'Cheers.'" It's at times like these that you must remember your loved one is anxious and sad. Be patient.

WINNING PLAYS: You should have a scheduled routine for each day that includes both definite activities and rest periods. Remember that your loved one needs structure, consistency, and repetition in each of his days.

Brainteaser #6: Dependency

This is a hard one, especially for mothers. It's so easy to fall back into a nurturing role, even if your child is an adult. But this can foster dependency, which will prevent your loved one from growing. The more dependent he becomes, the less responsibility he'll take on. Think of it. You'll have to make all his dentist appointments. You'll always have to do the food shopping. Your social sphere will become smaller. Like the cartoon baby in the classic "Who Framed Roger Rabbit?", you could have a whining, spoiled, cigar-smoking, sexually promiscuous "baby" on your hands.

WINNING PLAYS: Stop yourself before you do for him. Let him cut his own meat. Let him call the drugstore to renew a prescription. Take him shopping with you or when you make a social call. Have him join a support group where he can make new friends.

These are just a few of the "brainteasers" you might be forced to play. But remember: Take care of yourself. And keep a sense of humor. No, life isn't easy. It's full of surprises — and tragedy. But tragedy doesn't have to beget tragedy. You too can start that slow climb up; you too can recover from your loved one's brain injury and begin a new life.

Our journey is almost at an end, but to help you even further, we've included some of the most common questions people ask us. Join us for one last chapter.

CHAPTER FOURTEEN

QUESTIONS FAMILY MEMBERS COMMONLY ASK

"Beyond the bright searchlights of science,
Out of sight of the windows of sense,
Old Riddles still bid us defiance,
Old questions of Why and of Whence."

William Cecil Dampier-Whetham (1867-1952),
The Recent Development of Physical Science

Now that we've covered the different aspect of brain injury — the hopes, goals, and feelings of family and patient alike — you might be ready to ask some questions of your own.

Unfortunately we can't stand next to you as you read this book, but we can do the next best thing: answer classic questions that have popped up time and time again in our years of clinical experience. We hope the answers help you as much as they have helped those who first asked...

1. Will my loved one ever be the same?

This is a hard one, because the answer is tough: no. But can your loved one improve? Absolutely, yes. Good therapy, proper rehabilitation, and a positive environment can go far in helping your loved one realize his potential.

One of our patients had a severe brain injury when he was run over by a car while leaving work late one afternoon. His wife refused to believe that he would not come out of his injury intact, that he would be different from the man she had married. But the more she denied his injuries, the less help she could give — to her husband and to herself.

The trauma happened so fast. You saw the "miracle" of your loved one coming out of a coma. You saw him begin to walk and speak. Why wouldn't you believe that eventually his cognitive abilities would also completely return?

But you can't turn the clock back. What is, is. Instead of running from specialist to specialist looking for another "miracle," you must accept this new reality. With realistic hope, both you and your loved one will lead healthier and happier lives.

2. How long will the healing process take?

One of the more frustrating aspects of brain injury for families is the "wait-and-see" answers doctors give. These statements really aren't meant as brush-offs. Nor are they meant to be condescending. They are, unfortunately, very honest answers. The fact is, we often don't know how long the healing process will take. Everyone is unique, and predictors can only tell us so much. Even mildly brain-injured survivors can take from three to six months to improve. More severe cases need much more time than that. Healing takes time. As with broken arms and broken hearts, mending cannot be rushed.

3. Can't the doctor make the person I love wake up from a coma?

No. There is no magic or prince's kiss that can make a coma disappear.

Although drugs may be administered while the patient is in a coma, they are usually given to prevent seizures or spasticity, not to help the person awaken. (However, there is active research on drugs that might enhance emergence from coma.) Outside stimulation may not work, but it can't hurt. To this end, family members are encouraged to talk to the patient, hug or stroke him, show him photographs — in short, treat him as if he were awake. As you saw in Chapter Eleven, this is rehabilitation, and it can't start soon enough.

4. Do people in comas feel pain?

Think of a person in a coma as being under anesthesia for an operation.

She might groan or move her body in reaction to a cramp or a cringe, but she'll have no memory of that pain. And, unfortunately some painful procedures cannot be avoided for patients in a coma. Tracheotomy tubes, nastrogastric tubes, IVs, and catheters must sometimes be inserted, and this foreign apparatus can look especially painful to family members who have never seen any of it before.

5. My loved one's CT scan was normal. Why is he in a coma?

As we have seen in the beginning of this book, microscopic damage is not always picked up by CT scans, X-rays, or even the more sensitive MRIs. The patient may have diffuse axonal injury or brainstem damage that cannot be seen on the scans but keeps the patient in a coma.

6. Is my loved one malingering?

It's been our experience that most brain-injured patients actually try to minimize their deficits. However, if your loved one is dramatically acting out, throwing temper tantrums, and screaming, it's possible she is suffering from secondary psychological symptoms, in which case you should seek the advice of a brain-injury rehabilitation professional. In the meantime, try a reward system such as the one described in Chapter Eleven. Find enjoyable activities that you and she can share. Have her join a support group where she can meet others in similar situations. Be patient.

7. Does my loved one have to take her seizure medicine forever?

Probably not, but don't underestimate its importance: Seizures can cause additional physical injury. Anti-seizure medicine should be monitored. It's possible that its side effects might interfere with your loved one's rehabilitation. It's important to note that anti-seizure medicine should never just be stopped suddenly; abrupt withdrawal may actually cause seizures. Instead, the medication should be tapered off slowly under a doctor's full supervision.

8. How do I know when I need help?

Unfortunately, we can be so intent on aiding those we love that we neglect ourselves. If you become overstressed, you may be:

- Unable to sleep
- Poorly groomed
- Overwhelmed with guilt or feelings of unworthiness
- Feeling totally isolated and alone, with nowhere to turn
- Starting to use alcohol or drugs excessively
- Stricken with a sense of hopelessness — for yourself and the person you love

Remember, you must take care of yourself before you

can take care of anyone else. If you are experiencing any of these symptoms, speak to your case manager and seek out professional therapeutic help.

9. What about experimental therapies? Do they work?

Here's the run-down on some of the more popular fads:

• *Vitamins.* There is no concrete evidence to support the use of vitamin megadoses. If your brain-injured loved one is being given a nutritional supplement, it will contain all the vitamins he needs. And one multivitamin a day is generally all you need.

• *Special Diets.* Unfortunately, there's no such thing as "brain food." Nor is there any evidence that hair or nail testing is useful in diagnosing deficiencies in trace elements and/or minerals.

• *Hyperbaric Oxygen.* It's been tried for central nervous system diseases such as multiple sclerosis, but without success. If it doesn't work for MS, it is doubtful that it would work for brain injuries.

• *Brain Implants.* Although there has been experimental research on brain implants for patients with Parkinson's disease and stroke, it is a work in progress. Someday this may be routine therapy, but for now we will have to just wait and see.

HEADLINERS

THE PRIME OF MR. JAMES BRADY

It was a tragedy — it almost seemed as if history were repeating itself much too soon. Then-President Reagan had been shot, but it was his up-and-coming press secretary who took the brunt of the would-be assassin's bullet. That was in 1980. One and a half years later Brady had made vast improvement. Having escaped death from brain swelling and fluid building, Mr. Brady was already able to get around in a wheelchair. He could make jokes. Even his political acumen was intact. Why? Perhaps it was because he had such a strong personality. Perhaps it was the tremendous support he received. Perhaps it was his motivation to succeed in rehabilitation.

Today, James Brady is no longer a President's press secretary, but he and his wife, Sarah, successfully lobbied for the Brady Handgun Bill — and he is a role model and source of inspiration for thousands of brain-injured patients across the world.

• *Electric Therapy/Magnetotherapy.* Using electricity or magnetic fields to stimulate the skull does not improve anything, least of all cognitive function.

• *Acupuncture.* Yes, it does work to control pain, but acupuncture has yet to be proved an effective treatment for memory loss or cognitive dysfunction. Some new studies are suggesting it may help spasticity, paralysis, and motor function.

• *Chelation Therapy.* This is a process that uses chemicals to remove minerals, metals, and trace elements from the body. However, it's an unproved approach that could be dangerous. It's not performed by any reputable physician we know, nor is it supported by any recognized scientific organization.

• *Herbal Medicine.* Folk healers have long used herbs and roots to treat a variety of medical disorders, and herbs have become a booming business in today's "alternative medicine" world. But treating constipation or migraines is one thing. Developing memory, improving cognitive function, and changing inappropriate behavior are quite another. They are activities best managed by rehabilitation specialists.

10. My child was injured over a year ago, and the stress has been enormous. My family is falling apart. Where can we go for some solid help?

The Brain Injury Association has hundreds of support groups across the nation. They also have a directory that lists rehabilitation hospitals from coast to coast. The BIA also sponsors conferences, and has a wide range of research resources you can receive by mail. To speak to a real person and to receive real help, call their hotline: (800) 444-6443.

11. Why does my son see double? Will it go away?

The eyeball is connected to six little muscles that move it around in the head. These muscles are controlled by equally small cranial nerves that come out of the brainstem and go into the eye socket. The brain coordinates the movements of our two eyes so we don't see double. When a brain injury occurs, these cranial nerves can be stretched and sometimes torn; the brain is unable to do its eye coordination job. The result? Your son sees double, or two of things.

Usually, the stretching slowly heals and the eye muscles strengthen. In the meantime, you can help make your son more comfortable by putting a patch over one eye; this will get rid of the extra image. An optometrist or ophthalmologist can also put prisms on a pair of glasses to straighten out the images for the brain. These prisms are pasted onto the outside of the lens and easily changed as eye movements change.

Occasionally, surgery on the eye muscles is needed, but it is best to wait 6 to 12 months after the brain injury to see how things clear up on their own.

12. Why does my husband ignore the left side of his body? He doesn't recognize his left arm as his own. And he doesn't dress the left side of his body.

This phenomenon is called "neglect," and it can be a common symptom in right-brain injuries. In these brain-injured people, the left side of the world literally doesn't exist; it is "neglected." Your husband can see his arm or the mashed potatoes on the left side of his plate, but his brain ignores them.

Neglect seriously interferes with rehabilitation. It is hard to work on strengthening an arm that your brain doesn't know exists.

Fortunately, most symptoms of neglect show some improvement over time, but you must be patient. Until it starts to clear, you might feel that your husband's rehabilitation has stalled, even though your therapist is working very hard to reorient him to the left part of his world. His leg may be strong, but if he doesn't know that it is under him, he can't use it to walk.

To help ease your own frustration, don't forget to talk to your husband — and help him with his activities — from the side he recognizes. And always remember that rehabilitation works to compensate for "neglect."

13. My brain-injured daughter wants to drink a glass of wine or beer. Is it OK?

Ironically, alcohol is one of the major causes of brain injury. People who end up with a brain injury often had a drinking problem before the accident occurred; they shouldn't drink now — or ever.

Think of the effects of alcohol on the brain. It dulls your senses. Slows your reactions. It can cloud your judgment. In short, it creates problems you don't need, especially if you are already brain-injured and have trouble in these areas.

In our experience, we've found that your daughter will probably not stop asking if she can drink. Be prepared for her to ask you over and over again. Try to describe a situation to her: Would she want to go out to a business lunch with her former boss to impress him that she can handle her old job, only to order a glass of wine and become disoriented, irritable, or fatigued? Point out that she is already having difficulty with thinking, coordination, and behavior, and the alcohol will only make these worse. You are saying no because you care.

HEADLINERS

ROAD RAGE

Even if your reaction time and your coordination are in perfect running order, it still might not be a good idea for you to drive a car. If your temper is short and you are easily irritated ever since your brain injury, imagine how you might act if you were cut off by a teenager in a jeep? Or if you are driving behind someone who doesn't realize that the light has changed from red to green?

Behavior can be the limiting factor — and the reason not to drive again. We have one young man, an outpatient at HealthSouth RIOSA, who kicked out the windshield in a sudden fit of rage as his mother drove 65 mph on the highway!

---

14. I want to drive my car again, to go where I want to go when I want to go. Who makes the decision that I can drive?

The desire to drive again is one of the most common questions we are asked. Everyone wants to drive. Getting behind the wheel is assumed to be an American right when, in fact, driving is a privilege, a skill that needs to be learned.

In most cases of severe brain injury, your judgment and your ability to control your behavior and reaction time are not adequate enough to drive. Worse, you will most likely be unwilling — or unable — to see your deficits. Instead, you'll make the assumption that since you could drive in the past, you can do so now.

It frequently takes a driving test to make severely brain-injured people realize the reality of their situation.

Your therapist can check your knowledge of the rules of the road, and see if you react quickly enough:

- Can you press on a pedal fast enough when a light turns red in front of you?
- Can you put on the brakes if someone suddenly walks in front of your car?
- Can you stop "on a dime" if the car in front of you abruptly stops?

If you answer "yes" to this "pre-screening" quiz, a road test or driving simulator is still necessary to ensure your safety — and the safety of those around you.

15. My wife just sits around the house. It's as if she doesn't know where to start. Why can't she plan her day like she did before the accident?

It's called initiation, and it's a critical factor for success at home, at school, or on the job. It's the ability to get up in the morning. Get dressed. Get going and do what needs to be done. Beginning a project and turning it in on time. Starting to cook dinner so it's ready when the family comes home.

This ability to initiate action is fragile, and it is frequently lost with a brain injury. Your wife may really want to get out of bed or off the couch, but her brain can't send the message to begin, to plan, to actually sequence things in the correct order. She might want to make the bed, but her thoughts are jumbled. She wants to put the blanket on before the sheets are laid. She can't find the pillows. She literally can't get out of bed to make it.

You can help your wife by structuring and organizing her day. Make a list of what she needs to do and when she needs to do it. Set a timer to go off to remind her to look at the list, or call her from the office to remind her to do a chore. Break these chores down into simple steps and write them down. (Remember the steps in making a peanut butter sandwich in Chapter Eleven?) Try to set a regular routine so that things are done at the same time every day.

16. I can't believe how tired I am all the time. I never had to take a nap before. What can I do?

Fatigue is the number one complaint among our brain-injured patients. It is both a physical and cognitive problem. We all know the good feeling of being tired after a good workout or after a long, productive day. But, if you are brain injured, you get tired way before nighttime because everything takes more effort. It can be physically harder to walk, write, or propel your wheelchair; you use more energy.

It's also more difficult to think. It takes a great deal of concentration to even read a short letter or remember the steps in a simple recipe. Mental or cognitive fatigue can be more disabling because it is harder to recover from and to compensate for. You need to do things for shorter periods of time and you need to take frequent breaks in between.

Then there's the psychological aspect of brain injury which can be equally exhausting. It's difficult to accept the fact that you just can't do as much as you did in the past. And the harder you try to do the same things in the same way, the more frustrated you become, and the worse you will feel.

Ask your doctors about medication to counteract the fatigue. Some people respond well to stimulants such as Ritalin® or Cylert®. Others do well with such antidepressants as Prozac® or Zoloft®.

17. My grandmother was just diagnosed with an aneurysm that burst in her brain. Will she have the same symptoms as those who suffer traumatic brain injury?

Brain tumors or aneurysms in arteries that break can create similar symptoms to traumatic brain injury, depending on where the aneurysm was and whether or not surgery was needed. The blood, now free, circulates throughout the brain and the damage it does may involve both sides of the brain.

Isolated brain tumors tend to cause more localized problems, depending on where they take root and grow. A brain tumor in the front section of the brain will frequently cause problems similar to a traumatic brain injury: poor judgment, improper initiation, an inability to plan and follow through.

The same strategies and programs that are used in brain-injury rehabilitation will also work for people who have brain tumors or aneurysms.

18. I used to be able to read and do work with the television on. But now it seems as if any noise will distract me and affect my ability to get my work done. Why?

It is amazing to watch a teenager listen to music and do his homework or notice our coworkers carry on conversations while the phone is ringing and they are being paged. This is called "selective" attention and it is exactly as it sounds: Our ability to filter out what goes on around us and pay attention to only what is important at the moment.

Other types of attention:

• "Divided" attention requires us to keep track of multiple tasks at the same time. Remember when your mother cooked, stirring a pot on the stove and, at the same time, kept track of her children playing in the next room, as well as reading the headlines in the daily newspaper?

• "Sustained" attention is our ability to stick with a task. Can you sit and read a book for hours? Or complete your needlepoint pillow?

• "Alternating" attention allows us to quickly switch our attention from task to task: watching the road, glancing out the rearview mirror, turning on the radio, then watching the road again.

Brain injury severely affects our ability to pay attention, it's difficult to "filter" out those distractions, the conversation in the kitchen, the cars honking outside, the television. It's hard to concentrate on the task at hand.

Here's what you can do to help your attention span and keep distractions at bay:

• Turn off the television and the radio when there's a chore to do.
• Perform only one task or activity at a time.
• Create a quiet, distraction-free, and calm environment.
• Converse with only one person at a time.

- Avoid crowds.
- Outline what you plan to do — and when.

Our book is coming to an end; our time together is almost over. We hope these questions were some of the ones you yourself had been wanting to ask, or at least that they've given you food for thought. We know there's plenty on your mind.

THE FUTURE IS NOW

We firmly believe that brain injury, while traumatic, is not the worst thing that could happen. If our children were in a terrible accident, we would want to do everything possible to save them. We would want the emergency and intensive-care units to do everything they could to keep our children alive. We would rather have these children in a wheelchair for the rest of their lives, relearning new behavior, discovering old memories, and finding new cognitive skills and activities of daily life, than gone from our lives forever.

One of the mottoes of the Brain Injury Association is "Because life after head injury may never be the same." But it is life. It hasn't ended.

And that life can still be rewarding. It can still be dignified. It can still be hopeful. Long-term success is possible. At HealthSouth, we see proof of this every single day

A HealthSouth RIOSA patient wrote these words 13 years ago in a review article, words that still ring true, loud and clear: "One friend who told me that 75% of me was better than 100% of others she knew will never know how much she helped me."

It is our hope that this book has helped you. We hope you now have a better understanding of brain injury — its symptoms and its pain. We hope you feel you've had a short course in the rehabilitation process, that you now know and understand how brain injury rehabilitation works, and why. We hope we have given you some confidence, some "essence," that you can take away and that will keep you strong and accepting.

We hope we have helped you to find hope and a reason to go on.

That is success. And it's what brain injury rehabilitation is all about — the success of helping others.

In fact, that's probably what life itself is all about.

EDUCATION AND SUPPORT

American Heart Association
National Center
7272 Greenville Avenue
Dallas, TX 75231
(214) 373-6300
(800) AHA-USA1 (242-8721)
www.AmericanHeart.org

American Occupational Therapy Association
4720 Montgomery Lane
P.O. Box 31220
Bethesda, MD 20824-1220
(301) 652-2682
www.AOTA.org

American Physical Therapy Association
1111 North Fairfax Street
Alexandria, VA 22314
(800) 999-2782
www.APTA.org

American Speech-Language-Hearing Association
10801 Rockville Pike
Rockville, MD 20852
(800) 498-2071
(301) 897-5700 (Voice or TTY)
www.ASHA.org

Association for Children and Adults with Learning Disabilities
4156 Library Road
Pittsburgh, PA 15234
(888) 300-6710
(412) 341-1515
www.LDAAmerica.org

Association of Rehabilitation Nurses
4700 West Lake Avenue
Glenview, IL 60025-1485
(800) 229-7530
www.rehabnurse.org

Brain Injury Association
105 North Alfred Street
Alexandria, VA 22314
(800) 444-6443 (family help)
(703) 236-6000 (business office)
(703) 236-6001
www.biausa.org

HealthSouth
One HealthSouth Parkway
Birmingham, AL 35243
(800) 765-4772
www.HealthSouth.com

HealthSouth Rehabilitation Institute of San Antonio (RIOSA)
9119 Cinnamon Hill
San Antonio, TX 78240
(210) 691-0737

JCAHO (Joint Commission on Accreditation
of Healthcare Organizations)
One Renaissance Boulevard
Oakbrook Terrace, IL 60181
(630) 792-5000
(630) 792-5001
www.JCAHO.org

Joseph P. Kennedy Jr. Foundation
1325 G Street NW, Suite 500
Washington, DC 20005-4709
(202) 393-1250
www.familyvillage.wics.edu\jpks

National Stroke Association
7907 East Easter Lane
Englewood, CO 80112-3747
(800) STROKES (787-6537)
(303) 649-9299
(303) 649-1328 (fax)
E-mail: info@stroke.org
www.stroke.org

The Association for Persons with Severe Handicaps
29 West Susquehanna Avenue, Suite 210
Baltimore, MD 21204
(410) 828-8274
(410) 828-1306 (TTY)
(410) 828-6706 (fax)
E-mail: info@TASH.org
www.TASH.org

The Moody Foundation
704 Moody National Bank Building
Galveston, TX 77550
(409) 763-5333
(409) 763-5564 (fax)
www.moodyf.org

MEDICAL DEVICES AND ASSISTIVE EQUIPMENT

North Coast Medical
18305 Sutter Boulevard
Morgan Hill, CA 95037-2845
(800) 821-9319
www.ncmedical.com

Sammons Preston
P.O. Box 5071
Bolingbrook, IL 60440
(800) 323-5547
(800) 547-4333 (fax)
www.sammonspreston.com

Smith & Nephew
104 W 13400 Donges Bay
Germantown, WI 53022-8205
(800) 558-8633
www.smith-nephew.com

Superintendent of Documents
P.O. Box 371954
Pittsburgh, PA 15250-7954
(866)-512-1800
(202) 512-1800
(202) 512-2250 (fax)
E-mail: gpoaccess@gpo.gov
www.bookstore.gpo.gov

Documents available on disability law, health insurance
and the physically challenged

SOURCES

Alexander, Michael P., M.D., "Neurobehavioral Consequences of Closed Head Injury," *Neurology and Neurosurgery (Update Series)*, vol. 5, no. 20, 1984.

————, "Mild Traumatic Brain Injury: Pathophysiology, Natural History, and Clinical Management," *Neurology*, vol. 45, 1995.

Alves, Wayne M., Ph.D., and John A. Jane, M.D., Ph.D., "Mild Brain Injury: Damage and Outcome," *Central Nervous System Status Report*, edited by D. Becker, M.D., and J. Povlishock, Ph.D., National Institutes of Health, Bethesda, MD, 1985. Reprinted by National Head Injury Foundation, Inc., Southborough, MA: Article #85-021.

Barrer, Andrew E., Ph.D., and Douglas H. Ruben, M.A., "Understanding the Etiology of Brain Injury." Excerpted from *Readings in Brain Injury*, edited by Andrew E. Barrer, Ph.D., and Douglas H. Ruben, M.A. Reprinted by National Head Injury Foundation, Inc., Southborough, MA: Article #BIO84.

Barry, Philip, "A Psychological Perspective of Acute Brain Injury Rehabilitation," *Cognitive Rehabilitation*, vol. 4, no. 4, July-August 1986, pp. 18-21.

Batson, Meg, M.A., "Alcohol & TBI: A Problematic Pair," *Headlines: The Brain Injury Magazine from New Medico Head Injury System*, vol. 1, no. 1, Spring 1990.

Ben-Yishay, Yehuda, Ph.D., "The Role of Clinical Neuropsychology in Diagnosis and Rehabilitation," *Head Injury: Help, Hope & Information*, 3rd ed. Albany, N.Y.: The New York State Head Injury Association, Inc., 1984.

————, and George Prigatano, Ph.D., "Chapter 27: Cognitive Remediation," *Rehabilitation of the Adult and Child with Traumatic Brain Injury*, 2nd ed., edited by Mitchell Rosenthal, Ph.D., Ernest R. Griffith, M.D., and Michael R. Bond, M.D. Philadelphia: F.A. Davis Company, 1990.

Berrol, Sheldon, M.D., "Issues in Cognitive Rehabilitation," Archives of Neurology, vol. 47, February 1990. "Issues of Sexuality in Head-Injured Adults," *Sexuality and Physical Disability*, edited by David G. Bullard and Susan E. Knight. St. Louis: C.V. Mosby Co., 1981. Reprinted by National Head

Injury Foundation, Inc., Southborough, MA: Article #81-010.

Binder, L.M., and. J. Rattock, "Assessment of the Post-Concussive Syndrome After Mild Head Trauma," *Assessment of the Behavioral Consequences of Head Trauma*, edited by M.D. Lezak. New York: Alan R. Liss, Inc., 1989, pp. 37-48.

Blackerby, W.F., Ph.D., "Disruption of Sexuality Following Head Injury," Lecture handout materials.

———, *Head Injury Rehabilitation: Sexuality After TBI, HDI Professional Series on Traumatic Brain Injury* no. 10, edited by William H. Burke, Ph.D., Michael D. Wesolowski, Ph.D., and William F Blackerby, III, Ph.D. Houston, Texas: HDI Publishers, 1988.

———,"Disruption of Sexuality Can Have Traumatic Effect." Reprinted by National Head Injury Foundation, Inc., Southborough, MA: Article #87001.

Bond, M., "The Psychiatry of Closed Head Injury," *Closed Head Injury: Psychological, Social and Family Consequences*, edited by N. Brooks. Oxford, England: Oxford University Press, 1984, pp. 148-78.

Bond, Michael R., M.D., Ph.D., "Psychobehavioral Consequences of Severe Brain Injury," *Trends in Rehabilitation*, Bryn Mawr Rehabilitation Hospital Quarterly Magazine, Summer 1986. Reprinted by National Head Injury Foundation, Inc., Southborough, MA: Article #86-002.

Brigman, Cynthia, Carol Dickey, and Louise J. Zegeer, "Agitated, Aggressive, Patient," *American Journal of Nursing*, vol. 83, no. 10, October 1983. Reprinted in *Readings in Brain Injury*, edited by Andrew E. Barrer, Ph.D., and Douglas H. Ruben, M.A. Guilford, Conn.: Special Learning Corporation, 1984.

Brooks, D. Neil, Ph.D., "Chapter 12: Cognitive Deficits," In: *Rehabilitation of the Adult and Child with Traumatic Brain Injury*, 2nd ed., edited by Mitchell Rosenthal, Ph.D., Ernest R. Griffith, M.D., and Michael R. Bond, M.D. Philadelphia: EA. Davis Company, 1990.

Burke, Michael, "Reflections of a Brother," *Cognitive Rehabilitation*, vol. 2, no. 3, May-June 1984. Reprinted by National Head Injury Foundation, Inc., Southborough, MA: First Person Packet #P-007.

Burke, William H., with Mark Guth, Richard Guare, and Michael D. Wesolowski, *Head Injury Rehabilitation: An Overview*,

HDI Professional Series on Traumatic Brain Injury no. 1, edited by William H. Burke, Ph.D., Michael D. Wesolowski, Ph.D., and William E Blackerby, III, Ph.D. Houston, Texas: HDI Publishers, 1988.

————, with Michael D. Wesolowski, *Head Injury Rehabilitation: Applied Behavior Analysis in Head Injury Rehab*, HDI Professional Series on Traumatic Brain Injury no. 2, edited by William H. Burke, Ph.D., Michael D. Wesolowski Ph.D., and William F Blackerby, III, Ph.D. Houston, Texas: HDI Publishers, 1988.

————, with Richard J. Zawlocki, Michael D. Wesolowski, and Mark L.Guth, *Head Injury Rehabilitation: Developing Social Skills*, HDI Professional Series on Traumatic Brain Injury no. 9, edited by William H. Burke, Ph.D., Michael D. Wesolowski, Ph.D., and William F Blackerby, III, Ph.D. Houston, Texas: HDI Publishers, 1988.

Butler, Robert W. Ph.D., and Norman S. Namerow, M.D., "Cognitive Retraining in Brain-Injury Rehabilitation: A Critical Review," *Journal of Neurological Rehabilitation*, vol. 2, no. 3, 1988.

Byrne, Robert, *1,911 Best Things Anybody Ever Said*. New York: Fawcett Columbine, 1988.

Chance, Paul, "Life After Head Injury," *Psychology Today*, October 1986. Reprinted by National Head injury Foundation, Inc., Southborough, MA: Article #86-022.

Cytowic, Richard E., "The Long Ordeal of James Brady," *The New York Times Magazine*, vol. 131, no. 7, September 1981. Reprinted in Readings in Brain Injury, edited by Andrew E. Barrer, Ph.D., and Douglas H. Ruben, M.A. Guilford, Conn.: Special Learning Corporation, 1984.

Davis, Diana L., Ph.D., Manifestations of Neuropsychological Deficits Examples. Austin, Texas: Healthcare Rehabilitation Center, Lecture handout.

Deaton, Ann V, Ph.D., *Pediatric Head Trauma: A Guide for Families*, Cumberland Hospital, New Kent, Virginia. Austin, Texas. Healthcare International, Inc., 1987.

DiGiuseppi, Carolyn, M.D., M.P.H., Frederick P. Rivara, M.D., M.PH., Thomas D. Koepsell, M.D., M.P.H., and Lincoln Polissar, Ph.D., "Bicycle Helmet Use by Children: Evaluation of a Community-Wide Helmet Campaign," *Journal of the American Medical Association*, vol. 262, no.

16, October 27, 1989.

Dobkin, B. H. , "An Overview of Treadmill Locomotor Training with Partial Body Weight Support," *Neurorehabilitation and Neural Repair*, vol. 130: 157-165, 1999.

Dobkin, B.R., "Head Trauma," *New York Times Magazine*, October 9, 1988, pp. 50-51.

Eisenberg, Howard M., M.D. "Outcome After Head Injury: General Considerations," *Central Nervous System Trauma Status Report*, 1985, edited by D. Becker, M.D., and J. Povlishock, Ph.D., National Institutes of Health, Bethesda, MD. Reprinted by National Head Injury Foundation, Inc., Southborough, MA: Article #85-025.

Feld, Karen, "How Doctors Treat Severe Head Injury," *Parade Magazine*, March 18, 1984. (Reprinted in Readings in Brain Injury, edited by Andrew E. Barrer, Ph.D., and Douglas H. Ruben, M.A. Guilford, Conn.: Special Learning Corporation, 1984.)

Fisher, Jerid M., Ph.D., "Cognitive and Behavioral Consequences of Closed Head Injury," *Seminars in Neurology*, vol. 5, no. 3, September 1985, Reprinted by National Head Injury Foundation, Inc., Southborough, MA: Article #85-010.

Fordyce, David J., James R. Roueche, and George P. Prigatano, "Enhanced Emotional Reactions in Chronic Head Trauma Patients," *Journal of Neurology, Neurosurgery, and Psychiatry*, vol. 46, 1983.

Fralish, Kathleen, Ph.D., "Characteristics of Persons with Head Injury," *Innovations in Head Injury Rehabilitation*, edited by Paul M. Deustch, Ph.D., and Kathleen B. Fralish, Ph.D. New York, N.Y.: Matthew Bender, 1988, Frankowski, Ralph E. Ph.D., John F Anegers, Ph.D., and Steven Whitman, Ph.D., "Epidemiological and Descriptive Studies, Part 1: The Descriptive Epidemiology of Head Trauma in the United States," *Central Nervous System Trauma Report*, reprinted by National Head Injury Foundation, Inc., Southborough, MA: Article #85-019.

Fryer, Jeanne, Ph.D., and Kathleen Fralish, Ph.D., "Cognitive Rehabilitation," *Innovations in Head Injury Rehabilitation*, edited by Paul M. Deustch, Ph.D., and Kathleen B. Fralish, Ph.D. New York, N.Y.: Matthew Bender, 1988.

Furst, Charles, Ph.D., "The Neuropsychological Evaluation."

Excerpted from *Head Injury Symptoms: Brain Damage vs. Neurosis*, Los Angeles Trial Lawyers Association, 1984. Reprinted by National Head Injury Foundation, Inc., Southborough, MA: Article #BO484.

Goldberg, Stephen, M.D., *Clinical Neuroanatomy Made Ridiculously Simple*. Miami, Fla: MedMaster, Inc., 1979.

Goldstein, Felicia C., and Harvey S. Levin, "Epidemiology of Pediatric Closed Head Injury: Incidence, Clinical Characteristics, and Risk Factors," *Journal of Learning Disabilities*, vol. 20, no. 9, November 1987. Reprinted by National Head injury Foundation, Inc., Southborough, MA: Article #87-041.

Grafman, Jordan H., Ph.D., "Cognitive and Behavioral Sequelae of Head Injury," *Recent Advances in Head Injury: Annual Course #420*, American Academy of Neurology, Wednesday, April 19, 1989.

Guare, Richard, with Molly Samson, Mark Guth, Susie Warren, and William H. Burke, *Head Injury Rehabilitation: Developing the TBI Rehab Plan*, HDI Professional Series on Traumatic Brain Injury no. 4, edited by William H. Burke, Ph.D., Michael D. Wesolowski, Ph.D., and William F Blackerby, III, Ph.D. Houston, Texas: HDI Publishers, 1988.

Harvey E. Jacobs, Ph.D., "Chapter 20: Adult Community Integration," *Traumatic Brain Injury* (Comprehensive Neurologic Rehabilitation), vol. 2, edited by P. Bach-y-Rita. New York: Demos Publications, 1989, p. 331.

Hawley, Lenore A., *"A Family Guide to the Rehabilitation of the Severely Head Injured Patient."* Austin, Texas: Healthcare International, Inc., 1984, 1987. *HDI Professional Series on Traumatic Brain Injury, no. 8*, edited by William H. Burke, Ph.D., Michael D. Wesolowski, Ph.D., and William F Blackerby, III, Ph.D. Houston, Texas: HDI Publishers, 1988.

Hoine, Haskel, Ph.D., "Behavior Management of the Agitated, Aggressive Head Injured Patient," *Progress Report*, HealthSouth Rehabilitation Institute of San Antonio, Winter 1990.

————, "Psychological Adjustment to Disability," *Progress Report*, HealthSouth Rehabilitation Institute of San Antonio, Fall 1989.

Hopewell, C. Alan, *Head Injury Rehabilitation: Adaptive Driving After TBI*, HDI Professional Series on Traumatic

Brain Injury no. 5, edited by William H. Burke, Ph.D., Michael D. Wesolowski, Ph.D., and William F Blackerby, III, Ph.D. Houston, Texas: HDI Publishers, 1988.

———, "Practical Treatment Methods for Emotional Dysfunction," Lecture handout.

Howard, Michael E., Ph.D., "Family Adjustment to Head Injury," Lecture handout.

——— "Outcome from Head Injury," *Family Handbook of Head Injury*, Lecture handout.

———, "Recovery from Head Trauma by Levels of Cognitive Functioning," *Family Handbook of Head Injury*, Lecture handout.

Hutchinson, Ruth, M.S., and Terry Hutchinson, M.D., Ph.D., in collaboration with members of the Texas Head Injury Foundation, *Head Injury: A Booklet for Families*. Texas: The Texas Head Injury Foundation, 1983.

Johansson, B. P., "Brain Plasticity and Stroke Rehabilitation," *Stroke*, vol. 31, no. 7:223-230, 2000.

Kasowski, Janice Cortis, "Silent Epidemic," *First Person Accounts*. Reprinted by National Head Injury Foundation, Inc., Southborough, MA: Article #P007.

Kelly, J.P, and J.H. Rosenberg, "Diagnosis and Management of Concussion in Sports," *Neurology*, vol. 48, 1997.

Kline, Jeanette, "Knowing *What Was* Made It Difficult to Accept *What Is*," *First Person Accounts*. Printed by National Head Injury Foundation, Inc., Southborough, MA: Article #P-007.

Klonoff, Pamela, Ph.D., Kevin P O'Brien, Ph.D., George P Prigatano, Ph.D., Dennis A. Chiapello, M,S., C.C.C./S.L.P, and Marie Cunningham, C.T.R.S./C.R.T., "Cognitive Retraining After Traumatic Brain Injury and Its Role in Facilitating Awareness," *Journal of Head Trauma Rehabilitation*, vol. 4, no. 3, 1989.

Kraus, Jess F., Mary Ann Black, Nancy Hessol, Pacita Ley, William Rokaw, Constance Sullivan, Sharon Bowers, Sharen Knowlton, and Lawrence Marshall, "The Incidence of Acute Brain Injury and Serious Impairment in a Defined Population," *American Journal of Epidemiology*, vol. 119, no. 2, 1984. Reprinted by National Head Injury Foundation, Inc., Southborough, MA: Article #84-026.

Lemonick, Michael D., et al., "Glimpses of the Mind: What is Consciousness? Memory? Emotion? Science Unravels the

Best-Kept Secrets of the Human Brain," *Time Magazine*, July 17, 1995.

Levin, Harvey S., Ph.D., and Howard M. Eisenberg, M.D., "Postconcussional Syndrome," *Neurotrauma Medical Report*, vol. 2, no. 4, Fall 1988.

Levin, Harvey S., and J. Grafman, editors, *Cerebral Reorganization of Function After Brain Damage*, New York: Oxford University Press 2000.

Lewis, Frank, Ph.D., *Head Injury Rehabilitation: Developing Adaptive Work Behaviors*, HDI Professional Series on Traumatic Brain Injury no. 17, edited by William H. Burke, Ph.D., Michael D. Wesolowski, Ph.D., and William E Blackerby, III, Ph.D. Houston, Texas: HDI Publishers, 1988.

Lezak, Muriel D., Ph.D., "Living with the Characterologically Altered Brain Injured Patient," *Journal of Clinical Psychiatry*, 1978, Reprinted by the National Head Injury Foundation, Inc., Southborough, MA: Article #78001.

Liepert, J., H. Bauder, et. al., "Treatment-induced/ Cortical of Reorganization After Stroke in Humans", *Stroke*, vol. 6, 31:1210 1216, 2000.

Livingston, M.G., M.D. "Chapter 16: Effects on the Family System," *Rehabilitation of the Adult and Child with Traumatic Brain Injury*, 2nd ed., edited by Mitchell Rosenthal, Ph.D., Ernest R, Griffith, M.D., and Michael R. Bond, M,D. Philadelphia: EA. Davis Company, 1990.

Livingston, Martin G., M.D., M.R.C. Psych., and D. Neil Brooks, Ph.D., "The Burden on Families of the Brain Injured: A Review," *Journal of Head Trauma Rehabilitation*, vol. 3, no. 4, December 1988.

Lynch, William J., Ph.D., "Chapter 22; Neuropsychological Assessment," *Rehabilitation of the Adult and Child with Traumatic Brain Injury*, 2nd ed., edited by Mitchell Rosenthal, Ph.D., Ernest R. Griffith, M.D., and Michael R. Bond, M.D. Philadelphia: EA. Davis Company, 1990.

McMahon, B.T., and Flowers, S.M., "The High Cost of a Bump on the Head," *Business and Health*, vol. 3, June 1986, pp. 7-8.

McMcrea, M., J.R Kelly, et al., "Standardized Assessment of Concussion in Football Players," *Neurology*, vol. 48, 1997.

Miller, J. Douglas, M.D., Ph.D., and Patricia A. Jones, Dip. Phys., M.Sc., "Chapter 17: Minor Head Injury," *Rehabilitation of the Adult and Child with Traumatic Brain Injury*, 2nd ed., edited by Mitchell Rosenthal, Ph.D., Ernest R. Griffith, M.D., and Michael R. Bond, M.D. Philadelphia: E.A. Davis Company, 1990.

Mishkin, David, Ph.D., and Elizabeth Kampe, M.A., "Guidelines for the Management of Common Behavioral Problems With Post Trauma Patients." Reprinted by National Head Injury Foundation, Inc., Southborough, MA: Article #83-014.

Namerow, Norman S., M.D., Cognitive and Behavioral Aspects of Brain Injury Rehabilitation, *Neurological Clinics*, vol. 5, no. 4, 1987, pp. 569-83.

National Head Injury Foundation, *About Head Injuries*. South Deerfield, MA: A Scriptographic Booklet by Charming L. Bete Co., Inc., 1987.

National Head Injury Foundation, Inc., *Brochure*, National Head Injury Foundation, Inc., 333 Turnpike Road, Southborough, MA 01722.

National Head Injury Foundation, Inc., Newsletter vol. 9, nos. 3 and 4, Winter 1989-90.

National Head Injury Foundation, Inc., Questions About Traumatic Brain Injury (TBI), 1988. Article #84-005.

New York State Head Injury Association, Inc. "Head Injury Facts and Figures, General Characteristics," *Head Injury: Help, Hope & Information: A Family Guide*, 3rd ed. Albany, N.Y.: New York State Head Injury Association, Inc., 1984.

Nudo, R.J., "Recovery after Damage to Motor Cortical Areas," *Current Opinions in Neurobiology*, vol. 9: 740-7, 1999.

Nudo, R.J., "Remodeling of Cortical Motor Representations After Stroke: Implications for Recovery from Brain Damage, *Molecular Psychiatry*, vol. 2:188-191, 1997.

Nudo, R.J., E.J. Plautz, and G. H. Milliken, "Adaptive Plasticity in Primate Motor Cortex as a Consequence of Behavioral Experience and Neuronal Injury," *Seminars in Neuroscience*, vol. 9: 13-23, 1997.

Oddy, Michael, and Michael Humphrey, "Social Recovery During the Year Following Severe Head Injury," *Journal of Neurology, Neurosurgery, and Psychiatry*, vol. 43, 1980.

Parker, Roland S., Chapter One: The Hidden Epidemic," *Traumatic Brain Injury and Neuropsychological Impairments*, New York: Springer-Verlag, 1990.

Peterman, Bill, A Substance Abuse Program for Head Injury Survivors. Reprinted by National Head Injury Foundation,

Inc., Southborough, MA: Article #86-028.

Phoebus, Brenda, M.A., C.C.C./S.L.E, "Coma Stimulation: The Role of the Speech Pathologist, "*Journal of Audiology and Speech Pathology*, vol. 14, no. 2, Fall/Winter 1988.

Pollack, I.W, "Chapter 5: Traumatic Brain Injury," *Neuropsychological Treatment After Brain Injury*, edited by D.W Ellis and A.L. Christensen. Kluwer Academic Publishers, Norwell, MA: 1989, P. 420.

Prigatano, George P., "Emotion and Motivation in Recovery and Adaptation after Brain Damage," *Psychiatric Medicine*, vol. 7, no. 1, 1989.

————, "Psychiatric Aspects of Head Injury: Problem Areas and Suggested Guidelines for Research," *Neurobehavioral Recovery from Head Injury*. New York: Oxford University Press, 1987.

————, "Rehabilitation Interventions After Traumatic Brain Injury," *BNI Quarterly*, vol. 4, no. 2, Spring 1988,

————, and others, *Neuropsychological Rehabilitation after Brain Injury*. The Johns Hopkins University Press, Baltimore/London, 1985, p. 63.

————, David J. Fordyce, Harriet K. Zeiner, James R. Roueche, Mary Pepping, Beth Case Wood, "Neuropsychological Rehabilitation After Closed Head Injury in Young Adults," *Journal of Neurology, Neurosurgery, and Psychiatry*, vol. 47, 1984.

————, Mary Pepping, and Pamela Klonoff, "Chapter Seven: Cognitive, Personality, and Psychosocial Factors in the Neuropsychological Assessment of Brain-Injured Patients," *Clinical Neuropsychology of Intervention*, edited by Uzzell and Gross, Norwell, MA: Martinus Nijhoff Publishing, 1986.

————, Monte L. Stahl, William C. Orr, and Harriet K. Zeiner, "Sleep and Dreaming Disturbances in Closed Head Injury Patients," *Journal of Neurology, Neurosurgery, and Psychiatry*, vol. 45, 1982.

————, Kevin P O'Brien, Ph.D., and Pamela S. Klonoff, Ph.D., "The Clinical Management of Paranoid Delusions in Postacute Traumatic Brain-Injured Patients," *Head Trauma Rehabilitation*, vol. 3, no. 3, 1988.

Restak, Richard M., M.D., *The Brain*. New York: Bantam Books, 1984.

Rimel, Rebecca, W.R.N., N.P, John A. Jane, M.D. Ph.D., and

Michael R. Bond, M.D., Ph.D., "Chapter Two: Characteristics of the Head-Injured Patient," *Rehabilitation of the Adult and Child with Traumatic Brain Injury*, 2nd ed., edited by Mitchell Rosenthal, Ph.D., Ernest R. Griffith, M.D., and Michael R. Bond, M.D. Philadelphia: EA. Davis Company, 1990.

Roberston, I. H., and J. M. Muree, "Rehabilitation of Brain Damage: Brain Plasticity and Principles of Guided Recovery," *Psychology Bulletin*, vol. 125: 544-75, 1999.

Rosenthal, Mitchell, Ph.D., and Michael R. Bond, M.D., Ph.D., "Chapter 13:Behavioral and Psychiatric Sequelae," *Rehabilitation of the Adult and Child with Traumatic Brain Injury*, 2nd ed., edited by Mitchell Rosenthal, Ph.D., Ernest R. Griffith, M.D., and Michael R. Bond, M.D. Philadelphia: EA. Davis Company, 1990.

Sachs, Paul R., Ph.D., "Grief and the Traumatically Head-Injured Adult," *Rehabilitation Nursing*, vol. 9, no. 1, January/February 1984. Reprinted by National Head Injury Foundation, Inc., Southborough, MA: Article #84031.

Salazar, Andres, M.D., "Neurologic Sequelae of Closed and Penetrating Head Injury," *Recent Advances in Head Injury: Annual Course #420*, American Academy of Neurology, Wednesday, April 19, 1989.

Senelick, Richard C., M.D., "Angry Families and Angry Doctors," *Rehab in Review*, San Antonio Medical Gazette, November 27, 1996.

———, "Brain Trauma Has Many Causes, Complex Care," *Rehab in Review*, San Antonio Medical Gazette, May 8, 1996.

———, "Does Bubba Go Back in the Game?" *Rehab in Review*, San Antonio Medical Gazette, May 7, 1997.

———, "Head Injury: A Primer," *Progress Report*, HealthSouth Rehabilitation Institute of San Antonio, Winter 1990.

———, "Mild Head Injury: Separating the Wheat From the Chaff," *Progress Report*, HealthSouth Rehabilitation Institute of San Antonio, vol. 3, 1990.

———, "The Growth of Rehabilitation: RIOSA Stands Out," *Progress Report*, HealthSouth Rehabilitation Institute of San Antonio, Fall 1989.

———, "Malingering: It's a Tough Call," *San Antonio Medical Gazette*, December 25, 1996.

———, "The Use of Medications in the Head Injured Patient,"

Progress Report, HealthSouth Rehabilitation Institute of San Antonio, Spring 1990.

————, 'Whiplash' is No Head Injury," *Rehab in Review*, San Antonio Medical Gazette Focus Issue, July 24, 1996.

Shapiro, Kenneth, M.D., "Head Injury in Children," *Central Nervous System Trauma Status Report, 1985*. Reprinted by National Head Injury Foundation, Inc., Southborough, MA: Article #85-018.

Silver, J.M., S. Yudofsky, and R.E. Hales, "Chapter 10: Neuropsychiatric Aspects of Traumatic Brain Injury," *The American Psychiatric Press Textbook of Neuropsychiatry*, edited by Robert E. Hales, M.D., and Stuart C. Yudofsky, M.D. Washington, D.C.: American Psychiatric Press, Inc., 1987, p. 490.

Slaby, Andrew E., Ph.D., M.P.H., *Aftershock: Surviving the Delayed Effects of Trauma, Crisis, and Loss*. New York: Villard Books, 1989.

Sosin, David, David J. Thurman, et al., "Incidence of Mild Head Injury," *Brain Injury*, vol. 10, no. 1, July 1996.

Stuss, D.T., "A Sensible Approach to Mild Traumatic Head Injury," *Neurology*, vol. 45, 1995.

Tampa General Rehabilitation Center, Tampa, Florida, with Dana S. DeBoskey, Ph.D., and Karen Morin, M.S.W, *Head Injury: A Guide for Families*, HDI Coping Series no. 1. Houston, Texas: HDI Publishers, 1989.

————, Tampa, Florida, with Dana S. DeBoskey, Ph.D., Tyler Benyo, M.Ed., Connie Calub, M.Ed., Thomas Oleson, M.S., and Karen Morin, M.S.W, *Hiring the Head Injured: What to Expect*, HDI Coping Series no. 3. Houston, Texas: HDI Publishers, 1989.

————, Tampa, Florida, with Connie Calub, M.Ed., Dana S. DeBoskey, Ph.D., John Burton, M.S., Cathy Cook, M.S., Lisa Lowe, B.A., Dorothy McHenry, M.A., and Karen Morin, M.S.W, *Teaching the Head Injured: What to Expect*, HDI Coping Series no, 5, Houston, Texas: HDI Publishers, 1989.

————, Tampa, Florida, with Connie Calub, M.Ed., Dana S. DeBoskey, Ph.D., John Burton, M.S., and Karen Morin, M.S.W, *Life After Head Injury: Who Am I?*, HDI Coping Series no. 4. Houston, Texas: HDI Publishers, 1989.

Taub, E., N.E. Miller, et. al., "Technique to Improve Chronic Motor Deficit After Stroke," *Archives of Physical Medical*

Rehabilitation, vol. 74: 347-54, 1993.

Thickman, Mark, P.T., and John D. Ranseen, Ph.D., "Personality Changes Associated with Head Trauma: Implications for Rehabilitation Specialists," *Topics in Acute Care and Trauma Rehabilitation,* journal editor, Mary Kay Campbell, B.A., PT. "Head Injury" issue edited by Judith Verbanets, M.S., PT., vol. 1, no. 1, July 1986.

Thompson, Robert S., M.D., Frederick P. Rivara, M.D., M.P.H., and Diane C. Thompson, M.S., "A Case-Control Study of the Effectiveness of Bicycle Safety Helmets," *New England Journal of Medicine,* vol. 320, no. 21, May 25, 1989.

Traphagan, J.W.P., *Advocating for Funds.* Southborough, MA: National Head Injury Foundation, Inc., June 1988,

Traphagan, J.W.P., *Community Re-Entry.* Southborough, MA: National Head Injury Foundation, Inc., April 1988.

Tressler, Lance, ed., *Coma Assessment Scales with Stimulation Techniques,* National Head Injury Foundation, Inc., Article #8406. 1984.

Vogenthaler, Donald R., Ph.D., "An Overview of Head Injury: Its Consequences and Rehabilitation," *Brain Injury,* vol. 1, no. 1, Jul-Sept 1987.

Volpe, Bruce T., M.D., Topics in the Rehabilitation of the Head-Injured Patient, Lecture handout.

Wasco, James, M.D., "New Hope for Behavior Patients," *Headlines: The Brain Injury Magazine from New Medico Head Injury System,* vol. 1, no. 1, Spring 1990.

Weber, Lynn M., and Judith Verbanets, "Assessing Balance Performance in Moderate Brain Injury," *Topics in Acute Care and Trauma Rehabilitation,* vol. 1, no. 1, July 1986.

Weddell, Rodger, Michael Oddy, and David Jenkins, "Social Adjustment After Rehabilitation: A Two Year Follow-up of Patients with Severe Head Injury," *Psychological Medicine,* vol. 10, 1980.

Weinstein, Amy, with Elizabeth Moes and Margaret O'Connor, *Head Injury Rehabilitation: Management of Memory Disorders, HDI Professional Series on Traumatic Brain Injury* Houston, Texas: HDI Publishers, 1988.

Wesolowski, Michael, with Arnie Zencius, Richard J. Zawlocki, and William H. Burke, *Head Injury Rehabilitation: Developing Self-Control,* HDI Professional Series on Traumatic Brain Injury no. 14, edited by William H. Burke,

Ph.D., Michael D. Wesolowski, Ph.D., and William E.
Blackerby, III, Ph.D. Houston, Texas: HDI Publishers, 1988.

Wesolowski, Michael, with Richard J. Zawlocki, *Head Injury
Rehabilitation: Teaching Job Seeking Skills*, HDI
Professional Series on Traumatic Brain Injury no. 16, edited
by William H. Burke, Ph.D., Michael D. Wesolowski, Ph.D.,
and William F Blackerby, III, Ph.D. Houston, Texas: HDI
Publishers, 1988.

Williams, Janet, M.S.W. *What to Look for When Selecting a
Rehabilitation Facility: A Working Guide.* National Head
Injury Foundation, Inc., Southborough, MA: Article #85-011.

Wilson, Amani, Ph.D., *Clinical Applications of
Neuropsychological Testing: An Overview*, Wellesley, MA:
River Bridge Associates. Reprinted by National Head Injury
Foundation, Inc., Southborough, MA: Article #B1384.

Wolf, S.L., De. E.LeCraw, et. al., "Forced Use of Hemiplegic
Upper Extremities to Reverse the Effect of Learned Nonuse
Among Chronic Stroke and Head-Injured Patients,"
Experimental Neurology, vol. 104: 125-132, 1989.

Wood, R.L., "Chapter 10, Closed Head Injury: Psychological,
Social and Family Consequences, Brooks, N. (ed), New
York, Oxford University Press, 1984, pp. 195-220.

Ylvisaker, Mark, *Head Injury Rehabilitation: Head Injury
Rehab with Children and Adults*, HDI Professional Series on
Traumatic Brain Injury no. 12, edited by William H. Burke,
Ph.D., Michael D. Wesolowski, Ph.D., and William E.
Blackerby, III, Ph.D. Houston, Texas: HDI Publishers, 1988.

Ylvisaker, Mark, *Head Injury Rehabilitation: Management of
Communication and Language Deficits*, HDI Professional
Series on Traumatic Brain Injury no. 20, edited by William H.
Burke, Ph.D., Michael D. Wesolowski, Ph.D., and William F
Blackerby, III, Ph.D. Houston, Texas: HDI Publishers, 1988.

Zinner, Ellen, Ph.D., "Mother's Grief Reactions Studied," For
Your Information column in *Newsletter*, Winter 1989-90, vol.
9, no. 3 & 4, National Head Injury Foundation, Inc.,
Southborough, MA 01772, Mortality and Morbidity Weekly
Report, The Centers for Disease Control, June 10, 1997.

————, "What are the Options?" Compiled from interviews
with William Burke, Ph.D., John Fanning, Ph.D., Frank
Sparadeo, Ph.D., Allan Kraft, L.M.S.W, Jayne M. Wilson,
M.S.W, and Grace Smythe, *Headlines: The Brain Injury
Magazine from New Medico Head Injury System*, vol. 1, no.

1, Spring 1990.

———, "Up Close with Case Manager Sue Haley," *Progress Report*, HealthSouth Rehabilitation institute of San Antonio, Winter 1990.

———, "High Observation Unit," *Progress Report*, HealthSouth Rehabilitation Institute of San Antonio, Winter 1990.

———, "If This is Therapy, Why Are We Having So Much Fun," *Progress Report*, HealthSouth Rehabilitation Institute of San Antonio, Fall 1989.

———, "New Drugs Could Curb Brain Damage," *Headlines: The Brain Injury Magazine from New Medico Head Injury System*, vol. 1, no. 1, Spring 1990.

———, "Nurse Liaison Helps Smooth Transitions," *Progress Report*, HealthSouth Rehabilitation Institute of San Antonio, Fall 1989.

———, "Practice Parameter: The Management of Concussion in Sports." Report of the Quality Standards Subcommittee, *Neurology*, vol. 48, 1997.

———, "Return to Work," *Progress Report*, HealthSouth Rehabilitation Institute of San Antonio, Fall 1989.

———, "Trauma Happens to People: Adjusting to Disability," *Progress Report*, HealthSouth Rehabilitation Institute of San Antonio, Fall 1989.

———, *Some Symptoms and Characteristic Behavior Patterns of Those Who Have Suffered Traumatic Closed Head Injuries*, Institute of Physical Medicine and Rehabilitation, Peoria, Illinois. Reprinted by the National Head Injury Foundation, Inc., Southborough, MA. Article #84-007.

———, "Behavior Analysis: Treatment That Works for TBI." Compiled from *Applied Behavior Analysis in Head Injury Rehabilitation* by William Burke, Ph.D., and Michael Wesolowski, Ph.D., in *Rehabilitation Nursing*, vol. 13, no. 4, 1988, and Headlines: The Brain Injury Magazine from New Medico Head Injury System, vol. 1, no. 1, Spring 1990.

———, "Coma Intervention Tugs on Heartstrings," *Headlines: The Brain Injury Magazine from New Medico Head Injury System*, vol. 1, no. 1, Spring 1990.

———, "Emotionally Charged," *Headlines: The Brain Injury Magazine from New Medico Head Injury System*, vol. 1, no. 1, Spring 1990.

———, *Co-Treatment Outline*, HealthSouth Rehabilitation Institute of San Antonio. Lecture handout.

INDEX

ABOUT THE AUTHORS

RICHARD C. SENELICK, M.D., is the Medical Director at the HealthSouth Rehabilitation Institute of San Antonio (RIOSA). He also serves as Program Director of its Brain Injury program. A native of Illinois, Dr. Senelick completed his undergraduate and medical school training at the University of Illinois in Chicago. A neurologist who specializes in neurorehabilitation, he subsequently completed his neurology training at the University of Utah in Salt Lake City. Dr. Senelick has authored numerous publications, including co-authoring *Living with Stroke: A Guide for Families, Beyond Please and Thank you: A Disability Awareness Handbook for Family, Friends and Coworkers,* and *The Spinal Cord Injury Handbook.* Dr. Senelick is also is also the Editor-in-Chief of HealthSouth Press.

KARLA DOUGHERTY is a leading writer in the fields of medicine, health, and nutrition. She has authored or coauthored over thirty books, including *The Spark: The Revolutionary 3-Week Fitness Plan That Changes Everything You Know About Exercise, Weight Control, and Health* and *The Complete Idiot's Guide to First Aid Basics.* As the senior writer for HealthSouth Press, she has collaborated with Dr. Senelick on many books, including *Living With Stroke: A Guide for Families, Beyond Please and Thank You: A Disability Awareness Handbook for Family, Friends, and CoWorkers,* and *The Spinal Cord Injury Handbook.* She lives in Montclair, New Jersey.

"Getting People Back"
— The HEALTHSOUTH Rehabilitation Series

Getting people back... to work... to play... to living.® It has been the HEALTHSOUTH commitment since we first started taking care of people with disabilities and injuries. Now HEALTHSOUTH Press continues this tradition with "Getting People Back" — The HEALTHSOUTH Rehabilitation Series.

These books are specifically designed for people who need up to date, authoritative and easy-to-access knowledge about their problems. In a user-friendly, simple manner, these books, videos and study guides help educate patients and their families.

Through knowledge and education comes empowerment and the ability to do more than just "live" with a disability. These books provide the opportunity to exceed expectations and get people back.

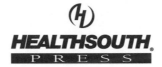

HEALTHSOUTH.
P R E S S

The HealthSouth Press Library is dedicated to helping people get back to their lives after trauma, an accident or illness. Our books demonstrate, in compassionate yet authoritative terms, how you and your loved ones can overcome a disability and live a full, rich life.

Utilizing the experience and up-to-the-minute technology of our vast network of rehabilitation hospitals and skilled physicians, therapists and health professionals, HealthSouth Press promises to show you a new and better way to adjust to a new life. Our books provide hope. Not false hope, but possible, viable and very real hope.

If you would like to order any of the books or video cassettes in our catalogue, please mail the order form to: HealthSouth Press, 9119 Cinnamon Hill, San Antonio, TX 78240. You can also visit our Web site at www.healthsouthpress.com

For additional information or to order by phone using Visa or MasterCard, please call 210 691-0737, ext. 300. You can also fax your order to 210 558-1297.

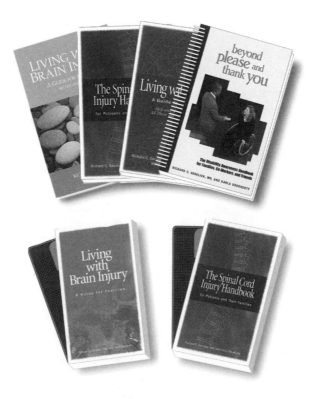

Order Form

For additional information or to order by phone using
Visa or MasterCard, please call 210 691-0737, ext. 300.
You can also fax your order to 210 558-1297.

QUANTITY   TOTAL COST

_____ *Living with Brain Injury: A Guide for Families*
      Second Edition ($14.95) $ _____

_____ *Living with Brain Injury: The Video ($19.95)* $ _____

_____ *Living with Stroke:*
      A Guide for Families ($14.95) $ _____

_____ *Beyond Please and Thank You:*
      The Disability Awareness Handbook ($14.95) $ _____

_____ *Beyond Please and Thank You:*
      The Study Guide ($3.95) $ _____

_____ *The Spinal Cord Injury Handbook ($12.95)* $ _____

_____ *Spinal Cord Injury: The Video ($19.95)* $ _____

                            Subtotal $ _____

                  Shipping (See rates below) $ _____

                        Sales Tax $ _____
                    (Texas residents add 7.875%)
                        Order Total $ _____

             ☐ MasterCard   ☐ Visa

Credit card # _____

Expiration date _____

Authorized signature _____

Ship to:

Name _____

Title _____

Address _____

City_____ State _____ Zip _____

Phone _____

Shipping Rates

$2.50 1 book	$7.50 6-10 books	$15.50 21-30 books
$4.50 2-3 books	$9.50 11-15 books	$20.00 31-40 books
$6.50 4-5 books	$11.50 16-20 books	$25.00 41-50 books

**Please call 210 691-0737, ext. 300, for rates outside the continental United
States and if ordering more than 50 books.**

Please mail order form to:
HealthSouth Press
9119 Cinnamon Hill
San Antonio, Texas 78240